EUGENICS IN JAPAN

EDITED BY **KAREN J. SCHAFFNER**

日本の優生学

カレン・J. シャフナー［編］

Kyushu University Press

All rights reserved. No part of this publication may be reproduced or transmitted in any form or by any means, electronic or mechanical, including photocopying and recording, or by any information storage and retrieval system, without the written permission from the publisher.

Copyright © 2014 by Karen J. Schaffner

Kyushu University Press
7-1-146, Hakozaki Higashi-ku, Fukuoka-shi 812-0053, Japan

ISBN 978-4-7985-0128-4

Printed in Japan

Contents

Prologue		*Karen J. Schaffner*	1
Introduction: Early Ideas of Race Betterment in Japan		*Karen J. Schaffner*	6

Part I Reception of Eugenic Thought in Japan

Chapter 1	The Birth of Genetics and Eugenics	*Yamazaki Kiyoko*	15
Chapter 2	Eugenics and Psychiatric Medicine	*Kitagaki Tōru*	34
Chapter 3	Eugenic Thought of Abe Isoo, Social Reformer in Japan	*Kawashima Sachio*	44
Chapter 4	"Good Wives, Wise Mothers" and "Racial Poisons" in Japan	*Karen J. Schaffner*	61

Part II Japanese Eugenics Connections

Chapter 5	Japan-U. S. Eugenics Connections	*Karen J. Schaffner*	71
Chapter 6	Nazi Sterilization Law and Japan	*Kawashima Sachio*	83

Part III Implementation of Eugenics in Japan

Chapter 7	Eugenics: Its Spread and Decline	*Chūman Mitsuko*	97
Chapter 8	Eugenics and Minorities	*Fujino Yutaka*	122
Chapter 9	Eugenics and Hansen's Disease Patients	*Fujino Yutaka*	131

Epilogue	*Karen J. Schaffner*	143
Chronology of Eugenics in Japan		147
Index		159

目　次

プロローグ……………………………………………カレン・J. シャフナー　1

序論：日本における優生思想の萌芽……………………カレン・J. シャフナー　6

第1部　日本における優生思想の受け入れ

第1章　遺伝学の誕生と優生学……………………………………山崎喜代子　15

第2章　優生学と精神医学……………………………………………北垣　徹　34

第3章　社会運動家　安部磯雄の優生思想………………………河島幸夫　44

第4章　優生学と女性……………………………………カレン・J. シャフナー　61
　　　　──「良妻賢母」が民を「民族毒」から守る──

第2部　日本優生学と欧米コネクション

第5章　日本と米国の優生学的コネクション……………カレン・J. シャフナー　71

第6章　ナチス断種法と日本…………………………………………河島幸夫　83

第3部　日本における優生政策の適用

第7章　優生思想の隆盛と退潮……………………………………中馬充子　97

第8章　優生思想とマイノリティ……………………………………藤野　豊　122

第9章　優生思想とハンセン病患者…………………………………藤野　豊　131

エピローグ……………………………………………カレン・J. シャフナー　143

日本の優生学関連年表………………………………………………………147

索　引…………………………………………………………………………159

Contributors

(in alphabetical order)

Chūman Mitsuko: Professor, Seinan Gakuin University, Department of Human Sciences, Division of Social Welfare ...Chapter 7
中馬充子：西南学院大学人間科学部教授。保健学（保健思想史）

Fujino Yutaka: Professor, Keiwa College (Niigata), Department of Literature, Division of Intercultural Studies ...Chapters 8, 9
藤野　豊：敬和学園大学人文学部教授（日本近現代史）

Kawashima Sachio: Emeritus Professor Seinan Gakuin University, Department of Law, Division of International Relations Law ...Chapters 3, 6
河島幸夫：西南学院大学名誉教授。政治学（ドイツ政治と宗教）

Kitagaki Tōru: Professor, Seinan Gakuin University, Department of Literature, Division of Foreign Languages, French Course ...Chapter 2
北垣　徹：西南学院大学文学部教授。社会学（知識社会学・社会思想史）

Schaffner, Karen J.: Professor, Seinan Gakuin University, Department of Intercultural Studies ...Prologue, Introduction, Chapters 4, 5, Epilogue
カレン・J．シャフナー：西南学院大学国際文化学部教授。社会倫理学（神学・アメリカ文化史）

Yamazaki Kiyoko: Professor, Seinan Gakuin University, Department of Human Sciences, Division of Social Welfare ...Chapter 1
山崎喜代子：西南学院大学人間科学部教授。生物学（発生生物学・生命倫理学）

Prologue

Karen J. Schaffner

> *Eugenics is the study of all of the agencies under social control that may improve or impair the inborn qualities of future generations of man, either physically or mentally.*
>
> Francis Galton

The above quote appeared in the masthead of *Eugenics: A Journal of Race Betterment*, published by the American Eugenics Society from October 1928 until February 1931. Noteworthy are the words "social control,"[1] "inborn qualities,"[2] and "future generations."[3] Eugenics was based on the supposition that heredity could be improved or impaired and promoted limiting the rights of individuals for the welfare of society, not only for that present time, but also for children yet to be born.

The theory of eugenics was one of several ideas which appeared in late nineteenth century England and began changing the ways people perceived human life and society. Influenced by Thomas Malthus'[4] ideas on population growth and natural selection, Charles Darwin[5] published *On the Origin of Species by Means of Natural Selection,[6] or the Preservation of Favoured Races in the Struggle for Life* (1859). Darwin's title implied that mankind could be divided into two categories—the favored and the unfavored. Herbert Spencer[7] postulated that only "the fittest" would survive in the struggle for life—again dividing mankind into the categories of "fit"[8] and "unfit."[9]

To these theories, Darwin's cousin and British statistician, Sir Francis Galton,[10] added "eugenics," a term he coined in 1883. Taken from the "Greek *eugenes*, namely good in stock, hereditarily endowed with noble qualities," it referred to

> the science of improving the stock[11]... which... takes cognizance of all influences that tend... to give to the more suitable races or strains of blood[12] a better chance of prevailing speedily over the less suitable (Galton 1883:24).

Galton had conducted hereditary studies of prominent British families which seemed to indicate that they were more likely than ordinary people to have offspring of repute. He concluded that greatness runs in families, and that traits of greatness—such as courage,

---

1. 社会統制　2. 遺伝性の素質　3. 将来の子孫　4. トマス・マルサス
5. チャールズ・ダーウィン　6. 自然淘汰　7. ハーバート・スペンサー　8. 適格者
9. 不適格者　10. フランシス・ゴルトン　11. 家系改良学　12. 血統

intellect and vigor, as well as wealth—are hereditary. His studies also noted that eminent families tended to have fewer children. For the good of civilization, he encouraged those families to increase their progeny, and less desirable families to decrease theirs.

Eugenics may have originated in Britain, but Galton's influence spread far beyond. In the United States, eugenics would help reform the working conditions for mothers and children, improve the mortality rate of infants, and curb the spread of infectious diseases. But it would also provide the "scientific" basis for racial segregation[1] and the segregation[2] and sterilization[3] of persons identified as "feeble-minded."[4] Restriction of immigrants[5] from Eastern and Southern Europe, as well as from Asia, was carried out to give greater advantage to the "more suitable races."

In Germany, eugenics was called *Rassenhygiene*, or "race hygiene."[6] The government took control of monitoring the health of its citizens, counseling couples whether or not marriage was advisable, and educating its young people in matters of health and hygiene. Hitler's "fitter Aryan race" would invoke eugenics as the justification for the extinction of Jews, handicapped, gypsies, homosexuals, and political opponents.

But eugenics would not be limited to Western countries; it would become a worldwide phenomenon. Associations, like the International Federation of Eugenic Organizations founded in 1925, were organized, and international congresses were held for the exchange of ideas and research. The definition of the "more suitable strains of human stock" was influenced by the various historical and social environments in which eugenics took root. Eugenics would be adapted to the purposes and goals of those who found it helpful for the "betterment" of society.[7]

Frank Dikötter's observations about eugenics are helpful in seeing how eugenics manifested itself in many different locales and times. "Eugenics was not so much a clear set of scientific principles as a 'modern' way of talking about social problems in biologizing terms." Thus, groups who were at cross purposes could embrace eugenics. He also notes that

> eugenics gave scientific authority to social fears and moral panics, lent respectability to racial doctrines, and provided legitimacy to sterilization acts and immigration laws. ... Eugenics promoted a biologizing vision of society in which the reproductive rights of individuals[8] were subordinated to the rights of abstract organic collectivity[9] (Dikötter 1998, 467-468).

The state, then, implemented polices and passed laws which infringed on the freedom and

---

1. 人種による分離　　2. 隔離　　3. 断種　　4. 「精神薄弱者」（知的障害者）
5. 移民制限　　6. 民族衛生　　7. 社会改良　　8. 個人の性と生殖に関する権利
9. 生成発展する集団体

the rights of some of their citizens for the good of the country. Some groups were forced to give up bearing children or living in the mainstream of society. Members of the "more suitable races or strains of blood" were encouraged to do their part in bearing many healthy progeny.[1]

Eugenics also took root in the thinking and policies of Japan.[*1] The development of eugenics in Japan is presented by Suzuki Zenji (1983) in his book on the thought and history of the eugenic movement. The ties of Japanese eugenics with fascism are found in Fujino Yutaka's book published in 1998. In *Yūseigaku to ningen shakai* [Eugenics and human society] edited by Yonemoto Shōhei, Matsubara Yōko has written a chapter on postwar eugenics in Japan. The timelines of Professor Hirata Katsumasa and Professor Katō Shūichi provide helpful overviews of Japanese eugenics and bibliographic sources. However, the Japanese language can be a formidable barrier to accessing these sources. In recent years, an increasing number of articles and books about certain areas of Japanese eugenics have been published. Many of these will be included in the references for this book. This volume will attempt to provide an overview of Japanese eugenics in English. It is our hope that this volume can serve as a bridge between English and Japanese. We will try to give some answers to such questions as: Who were the proponents of eugenics in Japan? In what circles was eugenic thought received? How was Japanese eugenics influenced by American and German eugenics? How was eugenic thought used to bring a "scientific" basis for government policies? Who were the targets of Japanese eugenic policies?

The introduction to the book gives an overview of the situation in Japan when eugenics was introduced and summarizes early "eugenic" thought. The first Part outlines the reception of eugenic thought by various groups of people—scientists, psychiatrists, social reformers, and women. Part two deals with American and German ties with and influence on eugenics in Japan. Part three looks at the application of eugenic thought to everyday life and some of the people and organizations which promoted eugenics. Also included are examples of how eugenics influenced governmental policies and which groups were affected by those policies.

This book is an outgrowth of an interdisciplinary bioethics study group at Seinan Gakuin University in Fukuoka, Japan. This study group has written a series of three volumes in Japanese dealing with the ethics of life [*Seimei no Rinri*]. The first volume, subtitled *Sono kihan wo ugokasu mono* [The things that motivate its norms], is a broad approach to bioethics from various viewpoints, one of which is eugenics. The second volume was subtitled *Yūseigaku no jidai wo koete* [Going beyond the eugenics era] and focused on eugenics in the United States, Germany, Japan, and Sweden. Research and

1. 健康な子孫

publication funds for these two volumes were made available by the university's Academic Research Institute. The third volume, subtitled *Yūsei seisaku no keifu* [The genealogy of eugenic policies], continued a focus on American, German, and Japanese eugenics. This volume was made possible by a grant from Seinan Gakuin University's Organization for the Advancement of Education and Research [西南学院大学教育・研究推進機構]. It should also be noted that none of these projects could have been completed without the collaboration of Kyushu University Press [九州大学出版会 Kyushu daigaku shuppankai]. Nagayama Shunji, editor at Kyushu University Press, patiently saw this volume through to publication. Also included in this last project was the reprinting of the journal *Yūseigaku* [Eugenics], published by Fuji Shuppan [不二出版]. Besides sixteen volumes containing the contents of the journal, there is a companion volume which includes a complete list of articles, an index of contributors, and a commentary written by Chūman Mitsuko.

Japanese names are written family name first, followed by the surname (given name) in Romanized form, using macrons for elongated vowels. Proper names that have been adopted into English, such as Tokyo and Osaka, are written without macrons. Publications, laws, and ideas will be given in Romanized spelling following the Hepburn method and with an English translation. For English readers who want to know the Japanese *kanji* and for Japanese readers who want to know the *kanji* or translation for people's names, titles, and key words, these are given in the lower margin of each page, designated by superscript numbers. Superscript numbers with an asterisk refer to notes given at the end of each chapter. A chronology based on events and publications discussed in this volume and an index can be found at the end of the text. Unless otherwise noted, quotations from Japanese are translations of the authors. Some historical terms, which may be considered degrading or discriminatory today, are used in the text from the standpoint of historical accuracy.

Notes

*1 Matsunaga Ei (National Institute of Genetics) has asserted that no eugenic movement has ever existed in Japan (Matsunaga 1968, 199). His article acknowledged a limited utilization of the postwar law for eugenic purposes, but did not address the wartime application of eugenics. Whether this is a case of selective amnesia or a specialized definition of eugenics, the following chapters should allow the reader to determine whether Matsunaga's assertion is valid.

References

Dikötter, Frank. 1998. "Race Culture: Recent Perspectives on the History of Eugenics." *American Historical Review*, 467-478.

Fujino Yutaka [藤野豊]. 1998. *Nihon fashizumu to yuseishisō* [日本ファシズムと優生思想 Japanese Fascism and Eugenic Thought]. Kyoto: Kamogawa Shuppan.

Galton, Francis. 1883. *Inquiries into Human Faculty and Development*. London: MacMillan.

Hirata Katsumasa [平田勝政]. 2004. "Nihon yūseiundōshi nenpyō (senzen hen)—shōgaisha no kyōiku fukushi to no kanren de—" [日本優生運動史年表（戦前編）—障害者の教育・福祉との関連で— A Chronological Table on Eugenics Movement in Japan before World War II] in *Nagasaki daigaku kyōikubu kiyō—kyōikukagaku—* 67 (June 2004), 21-28.

Katō Shūichi [加藤秀一]. 2002~. "Eugenics and Gender" < http://www.meijigakuin.ac.jp/~katos/ Eugenics.htm > < http://www.meijigakuin.ac.jp/~katos/Eugenics2.htm > < http://www.meijigakuin. ac.jp/~katos/Eugenics3.htm >

Matsubara Yōko [松原洋子]. "Nihon—Sengo no yūseihogohō to iu na no danshuhō" [日本—戦後の優生保護法という名の断種法 Japan: Postwar sterilization law under the name of Eugenic Protection Law] in *Yūseigaku to ningen shakai—Seimeikagaku no seiki wa doko e mukau no ka* [優生学と人間社会—生命科学の世紀はどこへ向かうのか Eugenics and human society—where is the century of life sciences headed], Yonemoto Shōhei [米本昌平], ed. Tokyo: Kodansha.

Matsunaga Ei [松永英]. 1968. "Birth Control Policy in Japan: A Review from Eugenic Standpoint [*sic*]" in *Jinrui idengaku zasshi* [人類遺伝学雑誌 Japanese Journal of Human Genetics]. 13:3, 189-200.

Suzuki Zenji [鈴木善次]. 1983. *Nihon no yūseigaku: Sono shisō to undō no kiseki* [日本の優生学—その思想と運動の軌跡— Japanese Eugenics: The Legacy of Eugenic Thought and the Eugenics Movement]. Tokyo: Sankyo Shuppan.

Yamazaki Kiyoko [山崎喜代子], ed. 2004. *Seimei no Rinri: Sono kihan wo ugokasu mono* [生命の倫理—その規範を動かすもの Ethics of Life: The things that motivate its norms]. Fukuoka: Kyushu Daigaku Shuppankai.

——. 2008. *Seimei no Rinri 2: Yūseigaku no jidai wo koete* [生命の倫理 2—優生学の時代を超えて Ethics of Life 2: Going beyond the eugenics era]. Fukuoka: Kyushu Daigaku Shuppankai.

——. 2013. *Seimei no Rinri 3: Yūsei seisaku no keifu* [生命の倫理 3—優生政策の系譜 Ethics of Life 3: The genealogy of eugenic policies]. Fukuoka: Kyushu Daigaku Shuppankai.

Introduction

Early Ideas of Race Betterment in Japan

Karen J. Schaffner

The introduction of Galton's "eugenics" to Japan was not the beginning of discussion about the need to improve the Japanese race and the ways to accomplish improvement. This chapter will look at the environment in which such ideas emerged, the impetus for such ideas, and several proponents of race betterment. Concern for the improvement of the Japanese race made Japan a fertile ground for the seeds of eugenic thought.

1. Meiji Japan: A Country in Transition

The late nineteenth century marked a major turning point in Japan's history. Apart from limited contact and trade with the Ryūkyūs (Okinawa), Korea, China, and the Netherlands, Japan had been virtually isolated from the rest of the world since 1639. Points of entry were limited, and foreigners kept separate from most people. Japanese were not permitted to travel outside the country, nor were foreign books allowed. However, those closed doors were opened, albeit reluctantly, in 1853 when Commodore Matthew Perry and his "black ships" from the United States arrived at the Edo port and demanded entry. Pressured into signing unequal treaties, Japan set about proving to the Western signatories that it was a civilized nation[1] worthy of a leading role on the world stage.

Changes swept across Japan. The center of government was moved from Kyoto to Edo (Tokyo). In what was called the Meiji Restoration[2] of 1868, a centralized government headed by the emperor replaced the ruling Tokugawa Shogunate.[3] The agrarian feudalistic society gave way to an industrialized capitalist society. Reforms were carried out in education, and in the military. Residents of the archipelago were encouraged to think of themselves, not as members of a certain clan or region, but as members of the nation of Japan. The Japanese word *for kokka*[4] [*nation*] is a combination the characters "country" and "home"—making each individual a member of the

---

1. 文明国　2. 明治維新　3. 徳川幕府　4. 国家

Japanese "family," whose head was the emperor.

Compared to other countries, Japanese often saw themselves as backward and behind the times. Their physical stature was also a cause of inferior feelings, as well as a reason why they were often considered childlike. They looked to the West to learn from them and incorporate the ideas, technology, and practices that contributed to their aims. By adopting "modern" practices and scientific thinking, they made preparations to be counted among the "civilized" nations of the world. The government adopted a policy of *fukoku kyōhei*,[1] a policy for enhancing the wealth and the military strength of the nation.

As the centralized Meiji government began nation building and developing a national identity, social Darwinism and eugenics were appropriated to galvanize a national consciousness which emphasized its fitness in the struggle for survival. Military success in wars with China and Russia signaled to the Japanese and to the world that it was a nation worthy of contention. At the same time, Japan distinguished its people from the neighboring Koreans and Chinese and the Okinawans and Ainu within in their borders.

In such an atmosphere, ideas were imported from the West. Westerners came to teach, and books were translated to introduce new ways of thinking. These ideas influenced how Japanese perceived themselves and how they felt the need to change in order to be counted among the powers of the world.

2. Input of Western Ideas

Foreign specialists were brought in to help Japan catch up with the West. One of the *Oyatoi gaikokujin*[2] [employed foreigners] was Erwin von Bälz,[3] a medical doctor from Germany, who came to Japan in 1876 under a contract to teach at the Medical Academy of Tokyo (later the Tokyo Imperial University School of Medicine). Bälz also had interest in anthropology and ethnology and encouraged his Japanese students to learn their history and culture instead of just trying to imitate the West. He supported the theory of a *Yamato* race,[4] which, although may have begun as an amalgamation of several races, had purified itself resulting in a strong race.

Zoologist Edward S. Morse,[5] who came to Tokyo the following year, lectured at Tokyo University. He was the first to introduce biological evolution[6] to Japan, not only to university students but in lectures to the general public as well. Morse, like Bälz, was interested in the origins of the Japanese race and culture. He conducted the first scientific archeological excavation in Japan at the Omori shell mounds in 1877. In these mounds were found pieces of pottery and scraps that gave glimpses of life in the Jōmon period.

---

1. 富国強兵　2. お雇い外国人　3. エルヴィン・フォン・ベルツ　4. 大和民族
5. エドワード・モース　6. 生物進化

He, too, provided materials for Japanese to investigate their origins.

These two are representative of the lecturers and technicians who came to Japan during the Meiji period, bringing knowledge from the West and encouraging Japanese scholarship. The translation of the works of other foreign scholars also introduced Japan to new ways of thinking, such as Lamarck's[1] inheritance of acquired characteristics,[2] Haeckel's[3] theory of evolution, Mendel's[4] laws of heredity, and Spencer's social Darwinism.[5] Japanese were also sent abroad to learn from the West.

3. Betterment of the Japanese Race

One of the entourage of envoys sent to the United States (1860 and 1867) and to Europe (1861-1862) to acquire new knowledge was Fukuzawa Yukichi,[6] founder of what was to become the first private university, *Keiogijuku*. His encounters with Westerners and Western civilization left him with the impression that Japanese were inferior, not only on the level of technological progress but also on a mental level. In his *An Outline of a Theory of Civilization*,[7] he contended: "... it has been only recently that we have realized Western countries are civilized while we as yet are not, and there is no one who in his heart does not admit this fact" (Fukuzawa 2008 [1875], 172).

Fukuzawa's writings on education show a connection between heredity and human ability and the acknowledgment of differences in that ability. Even at a time when the social system was changing to eradicate the class system, some people were from birth counted among the elite. No amount of change in the environment could improve what one inherited from one's parents.

Keio graduate and journalist Takahashi Yoshio[8] reflected his mentor's notion that Japan could not be counted among the "civilized" countries. In order to progress from a "semi-civilized" level, he asserted that improvement of the Japanese race was essential. In his 1884 essay *Nihon Jinshu Kairyōron*[9] [A Treatise on the Betterment of the Japanese Race], he proposed *kōhaku zakkon*[10]—mixed marriages between yellows and whites—as a strategy for race betterment. He suggested that such marriages between Japanese males and white females would improve the physique of the Japanese race, producing a population which could compete with the West (Suzuki 1983:32-34, 39).

In answer to Takahashi's suggestion that intermarriage with whites would improve the Japanese race, Katō Hiroyuki[11] offered a counterargument. He took issue with the premise that Japanese were inferior to Westerners and pointed out that the definition of "race" is vague. The process suggested by Takahashi would require a long period of time, and there was no assurance of the expected results. He argued that instead of

1. ジャン・バテスト・ラマルク   2. 獲得された形質   3. エルンスト・ヘッケル
4. グレゴル・メンデル   5. スペンサーの社会ダーウィン主義   6. 福澤諭吉
7. 『文明論之概略』   8. 高橋義雄   9. 『日本人種改良論』   10. 黄白雑婚
11. 加藤博之

improvement, intermarriage would so modify the race that a whole different race would be created, in effect destroying the Japanese race (Katō 1990 [1886]:33, 40-47; Suzuki 1983:35-38; Robertson 2005, 335-6).

In *Nihon fujinron*[1] [Treatise on Japanese women, 1886], Fukuzawa affirmed the value of Takahashi's marriage ideas, but also emphasized the need for personal improvement of Japanese parents. Improving one's way of life and environment are as important as heredity. Marriage is just one part of the equation. The chapter outline for Takahashi's treatise on race betterment shows his cognizance of the importance of multiple factors as well. Suzuki Zenji[2] gives the following chart illustrating the factors included in Takahashi's ideas about race betterment:

race betterment
[*jinshukairyō* 人種改良]
- heredity—marriage
  [*iden—kekkon* 遺伝―結婚]
- self-improvement
  [*shūyō* 習養]
  - physical
    [*shintai* 身体]
  - dignity of livelihood
    [*seikei no hin'i* 生計の品位]

(Suzuki 1983, 44; Takahashi 1884, i)

The dispute between Takahashi and Katō was finally settled by Bälz, who in a lecture entitled "*Nihon jinshukairyōron*"[3] [Theory for betterment of the Japanese race], commented on the arguments of the two men (Bälz 1886). About Takahashi's self-improvement (physical training along with decent living), Bälz voiced his agreement, saying he had made the same point in a lecture three years earlier. But he disagreed with him on a separate point: "I cannot agree with the importance he places on achieving race improvement through interracial marriage." Bälz further stated that Europeans would find this a truly "strange notion." Predicting whether a new race by means of mixed marriage would be superior or inferior is "an uncertainty." Then, while introducing examples of the results of interracial marriages in various other countries, he emphasized that carrying out such a plan would be very dangerous. Bälz sided with Katō, asserting that Takahashi's improvement plan was a most ominous one and that it was not a genuine improvement, but rather race transformation. Concerning Katō's and Takahashi's insistence that Japanese had no hope to win in competition with Western races in the future struggle for survival, Bälz voiced a strong denial. In 1885, just before Bälz'

---

1. 『日本婦人論』　　2. 鈴木善次　　3. 『日本人種改良論』

lecture, FukuzawaYukichi's *"Datsu a ron"*[1] [On departure from Asia] was released. According to this theory, he declined association with Chinese and Koreans—"the undesirable friends of East Asia," asserting that Japanese should "get rid of them and have contact with Westerners" instead. We can surmise that Bälz' comments that Chinese would not likely desire marriage with Japanese come from the context of Fukuzawa's "leave Asia, enter Europe" thinking.

Bälz' comments from his "Theory for the Betterment of the Japanese race" show that his ideas were based on an entirely different point of view than that of Takahashi and Katō. First, it is impossible to determine from one's physique whether or not one is in frail health, therefore it cannot be concluded that Japanese are frail. Secondly, because many Japanese people enjoy robust health and are hard-working, there is no reason to be afraid of competition in the fight for survival. Finally, frail health is more often found in the upper levels of society. Bälz pointed out that it is important to provide education concerning a correct, appropriate lifestyle and give consideration to heredity in selecting one's spouse. Above all, the viewpoint from Bälz' theory that must be regarded as most important is the warning that "doing uncertain things that cannot be predicted is very dangerous."

In 1892 Herbert Spencer provided words of advice concerning this issue at the request of the prime minister's aide, Kaneko Kentarō. His letter was reprinted in America's Eugenics Record Office[2] publication, *Eugenical News*:

> There is abundant proof, alike furnished by the intermarriages of human races and by the interbreeding of animals, that when the varieties mingled diverge beyond a certain slight degree the result is inevitably a bad one in the long run.... The consequence is that, if you mix the constitution of two widely divergent varieties which have severally become adapted to widely divergent modes of life, you get a constitution which is adapted to the mode of life of neither—a constitution which will not work properly, because it is not fitted for any set of conditions whatever. By all means, therefore, peremptorily interdict marriages of Japanese with foreigners. (Spencer 1892)

Spencer reiterates Katō's fear that miscegenation[3] would have a negative effect on the improvement of the Japanese race.

Takahashi had introduced Galton's *Hereditary Genius*[4] (1865) in the second chapter of his treatise on race betterment (Suzuki 1983 39-40). Galton studied men of reputation—judges, statesmen, commanders, scientists, poets, musicians, etc.—with the

---

1.「脱亜論」 2. 優生記録局 3. 異人種間結婚 4.『天才と遺伝』

intent of establishing his hypothesis that creative and intellectual abilities are hereditary. Galton's ideas are reflected in Takahashi's and Fukuzawa's writings which discuss how to improve the Japanese race. Galton had not yet coined the term "eugenics," but eugenic thought was already taking shape in his thinking, as well as in the ideas of race betterment in Japan. Subsequent chapters will show how and where eugenics took root in Japan's thinking and how it was applied.

References

Ameda Ei'ichi [雨田英一]. 2000. "Fukuzawa Yukichi no 'Maruhadaka no kyōsō' to 'Jinshu kairyō' no shisō" [福沢諭吉の「丸裸の競走」と「人種改良」の思想 Fukuzawa Yukichi's Ideas on "stark-naked competition" and "race betterment"] in *Tōyōbunkakenkyū* 2 (Mar.), 385-418.

Fukuzawa Yukichi [福澤諭吉]. 2008 [1875]. *An Outline of a Theory of Civilization* [文明論の概略 Bunmeiron no gairyaku], David A. Dilworth & G. Cameron Hurst, III, trans. Tokyo: Keio University Press.

———. 2003 [1888]. *Nihon fujinron* [日本婦人論 Treatise on Japanese women], Nishizawa Naoko, ed. Tokyo: Keio University Press.

———. 2003 [1896]. "Jinshukairyō" [人種改良 Race betterment] in *Fukuō hyakuwa* [福翁百話 Collection of 100 essays by Fukuzawa], Hattori Reijirō, ed. Tokyo: Keio University Press.

Katō Hiroyuki [加藤弘之]. 1990 [1886]. "Nihon jinshu kairyō no ben" [日本人種改良ノ弁 Discussion of the betterment of the Japanese race] in *Katō Hiroyuki Monjo* [Collected Writings of Katō Hiroyuki] Ueda Katsumi, et al., ed., 3:33-47. Tokyo: Dohosha Shuppan.

Macfarlane, Alan. 2002. "Yukichi Fukuzawa and the Making of the Modern World." ⟨http://www.alanmacfarlane.com/TEXTS/FUKUZAWA_final.pdf⟩

Morris-Suzuki, Teresa. 1998. "Debating Racial Science in Wartime Japan" in *Osiris*, 13:354-375.

Nishikawa, Shunsaku. 1991. "Profiles of educators: Fukuzawa Yukichi (1835-1901)" in *Prospects* 21:2, 287-296.

Robertson, Jennifer. 2005. "Biopower: Blood, Kinship, and Eugenic Marriage" in *A Companion to the Anthropology of Japan*, Jennifer Robertson, ed. Malden, MA: Blackwell Publishing.

———. 2002. "Blood Talks: Eugenic Modernity and the Creation of New Japanese" in *History and Anthropology* 13:3, 191-216.

Spencer, Herbert. 1892. "Herbert Spencer's Advice to Japan" in *Eugenical News* 11:11 (1926), 168-169.

Suzuki Zenji [鈴木善次]. 1983. *Nihon no yūseigaku: sono shisō to undō no kiseki* [日本の優生学―その思想と運動の軌跡 Japanese Eugenics: the legacy of eugenic thought and the eugenics movement]. Tokyo: Sankyo Shuppan.

Takahashi Yoshio [高橋義雄]. 1884. *Nihon jinshu kaizōron* [日本人種改造論 Treatise on the

Improvement of the Japanese Race]. Tokyo: Ishikawa Hanjirō. 〈kindai.ndl.go.jp/info:ndljp/pid/832935〉

Weiner, Michael. 1997. "The Invention of Identity: Race and Nation in Pre-War Japan," in *The Construction of Racial Identities in China and Japan: Historical and Contemporary Perspectives*, Frank Dikötter, ed., 96-117. Honolulu: University of Hawai'i Press.

Part I

Reception of Eugenic Thought in Japan

Chapter 1   *The Birth of Genetics and Eugenics*

Yamazaki Kiyoko

*I*n the economic infrastructure of each feudal clan of Edo era Japan, stable increase of agricultural products was of vital importance. Even in the early Edo period, more than a hundred varieties of rice plants, Japan's staple food, had already been created. Furthermore, publications in which characteristics and cultivation methods of various agricultural species and even methods of selective breeding[1] were given, became popular by the middle of Edo era. Later professional breeders in horticulture and animal husbandry developed breeds of morning glories, camellias, Japanese rhodea, silkworms, and domestic fowls (Kihara 1972, 275-298).

From 1639 to 1854, the Edo Shogunate adopted a national isolation policy, strictly controlling trade and communication with the outside world. During this time, Japanese scholars had very limited contact with foreigners and their knowledge. The one place they were able to study leading edge science and technology was a controlled area in Nagasaki called "Dejima,"[2] where a few European researchers and medical doctors were authorized to enter and live (Bartholomew 1989). The Meiji government, however, opened the country to the world. On the basis of policies to promote industry and increase wealth and military power,[3] every possible effort was made to learn Western scientific and social ideas. At this time when Japanese were voraciously absorbing knowledge from overseas, such ideas as Charles Darwin's[4] evolutionary theory,[5] Francis Galton's[6] eugenics,[7] and Herbert Spencer's[8] social Darwinism[9] were introduced.

1. The Introduction of Evolutionary Theory, Social Darwinism, and Eugenics

In April of 1877, the Meiji government established "Tokyo University"[10] as the first university in Japan by consolidating two colleges from the Edo Shogunate—Tokyo Kaisei Gakkō and Tokyo Medical School. Tokyo University established a Department of Biology in the Faculty of Science, which was divided into the Department of Botany and the Department of Zoology two years later. Tokyo University became "Tokyo

1. 品種改良　2. 出島　3. 富国強兵　4. チャールズ・ダーウィン　5. 進化論
6. フランシス・ゴルトン　7. 優生学　8. ハーバート・スペンサー
9. 社会ダーウィニズム　10. 東京大学

Imperial University" in 1897. By 1939, a total of nine imperial universities, including ones in Seoul and Taipei, and six national higher normal schools were established.

As faculty for these schools, some foreigners were hired. In 1877, Edward Sylvester Morse[1] was invited to be the first zoological professor of the Biological Department of Tokyo University. He had been a student of Louis Agassiz,[2] professor of natural history at Harvard University (Ueno 1988a, 77-85). The first botanical professor of Tokyo University was Yatabe Ryōkichi,[3] who had studied at Cornell University in the United States. He returned to Japan to join a staff of fifteen professors in the College of Science, twelve of whom were foreigners (Ueno 1988b, 86-93).

Morse enthusiastically taught evolutionary theory in Japan. In October 1877, he gave the first public lecture on Darwin's evolutionary theory in Japan in front of an audience of more than five hundred, including students, teachers, and ordinary people (Morse 1990, 339-340). In 1883, Ishikawa Chiyomatsu,[4][*1] who was a student of Morse in 1879, published the contents of the lectures under the title *Dōbutsu shinka ron*[5] [Evolutionary theory of animals].

Morse advocated the organization of an academic scientific society and established the Biological Society of Tokyo University[6] with Yatabe in 1878. This society separated into the Botanical Society of Tokyo[7] (1882) with *The Botanical Magazine*[8] (1887) and the Zoological Society of Tokyo[9] (1885) with *The Zoological Magazine*[10] (1888). Although Morse's stay was only two years, he laid the foundation for Japanese biology, which developed to a level comparable with that of biology research overseas.

Prior to Morse, a German teacher named Franz M. Hilgendorf,[11] who was a teacher at the Tokyo Medical School in 1873, had introduced evolutionary theory in his lecture. His student, Matsubara Shin'nosuke[12] described it in his 18-page booklet, *Seibutsu shinron*[13] [New theory of life] in 1879. Some of Darwin's original works were also translated during this period.[*2] In 1881, Kōzu Senzaburō,[14] a music educator, translated part of *The Descent of Man*[15] and published it as *Jinsoron*[16] [Human descent]. Izawa Shūji[17] was an educator who was sent to U. S. with Kōzu in 1875-1878 by the Ministry of Education to investigate the teacher training course. While there, he came in contact with Darwinism and intended to translate *The Origin of the Species*, but started with Thomas H. Huxley's *Origin of the species*[18] (Huxley 1863) instead. Ten years later, his translation was published as *Shinka genron*[19] [The principles of evolution]. He became the principal of Tokyo Higher Normal School, played a key role in educational administration, and promoted the adoption of the idea of social Darwinism into his work in Japan and East Asia. A translation of Darwin's book was published in 1896 as *Seibutsushigen ichimei shugenron*[20] [The origin of living things or the origin of species]

1. エドワード・S. モース　　2. ルイ・アガシー　　3. 矢田部良吉　　4. 石川千代松
5. 『動物進化論』　　6. 東京大学生物学会　　7. 東京植物学会　　8. 『植物学雑誌』
9. 東京動物学会　　10. 『動物学雑誌』　　11. フランツ・M. ヒルゲンドルフ　　12. 松原新之介
13. 『生物新論』　　14. 神津専三郎　　15. 『人間の由来』　　16. 『人祖論』　　17. 伊澤修二
18. 『種の起源』（トーマス・H. ハックスリー）　　19. 『進化新説』　　20. 『生物始源一名種源論』

by 28-year-old philosopher Tachibana Senzaburō,[1] who had been sent to study in Europe by the Imperial Household Agency.

The influence of social Darwinism deeply penetrated Japanese society's political and educational thinking. Herbert Spencer's *Education*[2] was translated by Seki Shinpachi,[3] published by the Ministry of Education as *Shishi kyōikuron*[4] [Spencer's education theory] and was widely read. Fukuzawa Yukichi,[5] a leader of modern thinking, adopted Spencer's *Education* as a university textbook in English (Inatomi 1956, 345-346). Katō Hiroyuki[6] played a central role in the government as president of Tokyo University and as a member of the House of Peers and the Privy Council. Like Fukuzawa, he was originally a natural rights activist, but, under the influence of Spencer and Darwin, he began to emphasize the struggle and competition in society and education (Xu 1991).

Ikeda Shigenori,[7] who was a leader the Eugenic Exercise/Movement,[*3] wrote that Galton's name appeared in the early Meiji period (Ikeda 1926, 4), but this reference is unclear. Fukuzawa introduced Galton's *Hereditary Genius*[8] in his *Jijishōgen*[9] [Commentary on current problems] and advocated eugenic arguments (Fukuzawa 1881, 225). After that, he continued promoting the application of eugenic policy (Ameda 1999). Galton's *Hereditary Genius*[10] was translated into Japanese as *Tensai to iden* [Genius and Heredity] by psychologist Haraguchi Tsuruko[11] in 1916, who was the first Japanese woman to receive a Ph.D. degree from Columbia University.

Before the turn of the century, the theories and writings of Darwin, Huxley, Spencer, and Galton were introduced into Japan in lectures and translations, but it is of note that biologists made no translations of original works on social Darwinism or eugenics.

2. Introduction of Mendel's Laws and Toyama Kametarō as a Pioneer of Genetics

As far as I have determined, the first mention of Mendel's laws[12] in scientific journals was in the 1903 issue of *The Zoological Magazine*. Kuwano Hisataka,[13] a 1901 graduate of Tokyo Imperial University's Faculty of Zoology and later professor in the Tokyo women's normal school, translated an article by A. D. Darbishire[14] in which Mendel's laws were mentioned (Darbishire 1902).

Miyake Kiichi (later professor at Tokyo Imperial University's College of Agriculture)[15] reported on a 1903 committee meeting of the International Botanist Association in Leiden with Fujii Kenjirō[16] and their visit with Hugo M. de Vries,[17] one of those who rediscovered Mendel's laws in 1900. Although Miyake didn't mention

1. 立花銑三郎   2. 『教育論』(H. スペンサー)   3. 尺振八   4. 『斯氏教育論』
5. 福澤諭吉   6. 加藤弘之   7. 池田林儀   8. 『遺伝的天才』   9. 『時事小言』
10. 『天才と遺伝』   11. 原口鶴子   12. メンデルの法則   13. 桑野久任
14. アーサー・D. ダルビシャー   15. 三宅驥一   16. 藤井健次郎
17. ユーゴ・ド・フリース

Mendel's laws directly, he certainly knew of them. The term "Mendel's laws" appeared in an article by Shibata Keita,[1] who was later professor of botany at Tokyo Imperial University (Shibata 1904, 127). Miyoshi Manabu[2] and Ikeno Sei'ichiro[3] published technical botanical books in 1906 in which Mendel's laws were mentioned in detail (Miyoshi 1906, 640-655; Ikeno 1906, 61-70).

The first practical application of Mendel's laws of heredity was in the silk industry. Around 1900, genetic research of the silkworm[4] had already begun in Japan by agronomist Toyama Kametarō,[5] associate professor at Tokyo Imperial University's College of Agriculture from 1902. In a monograph published in 1906, he demonstrated that the heredity of the color of silkworm eggs, larval speckles, and the colors of the cocoon followed Mendel's laws (Toyama 1906; Onaga 2010, 215-64), providing the first proof that Mendel's laws were also applicable to insects. At the same time, he discovered maternal inheritance[6] and the existence of heredity that disagreed with Mendel's laws, and showed the principle of hybrid vigor.[7] In a sericulture[8] textbook, his explanation of heredity included Mendel's laws (Toyama 1909, 278-304). When the Japanese government passed a law in 1894 founding national agriculture experimental stations[9] in seven locations, researchers and engineers used Mendel's laws to develop new hybrid strains of rice and wheat (Matsubara 2006, 92).

During those years, there were no articles to be found about eugenics. However, Japanese biologists gradually became interested in eugenics because of the news of Galton's death, the 1st International Congress of Eugenics,[10] as well as an increase in genetic subjects in articles of *The Zoological Magazine* after 1908, like Ōshima Hiroshi's[11] "*Iden ni tsuite*" [On heredity] in 1909.

3. Biologists, Agronomists, and Eugenics in Meiji Japan

As noted above, Ishikawa Chiyomatsu, having studied under Morse and Weismann, was an avid promoter of Darwin's evolutionary theory. With his training in natural history, he constructed the foundation for Japanese biology and genetics. He also participated a role in the organization of the Genetics Society[12] of Japan in 1920, the Japan Eugenics Society in 1924, the Japan Eugenic Education Society[13] in 1926, and the Japan Society of Race Hygiene[14] in 1930.

In his book *Ningen no shinka*[15] [Human evolution], Ishikawa asserted that the improvement of both the germ plasm and the environment were necessary to create good human beings. Furthermore, he seemed to keep a levelheaded distance from Galton's eugenics:

1. 柴田圭太　2. 三好学　3. 池野成一郎　4. カイコ（蚕）　5. 外山亀太郎
6. 母性遺伝　7. 雑種強勢　8. 養蚕学　9. 国立農業試験場
10. 第一回国際優生学会　11. 大島廣　12. 日本優生学協会　13. 日本優生教育学会
14. 日本民族衛生学会　15. 『人間の進化』

I have heard that Pearl[1]*[4] looked into the heritage of great people listed in the British Encyclopedia, excluding politicians and military men, and made a list more than a page long of great people whose parents were obscure ordinary people. ... It is well known that in *Hereditary Genius* Galton listed many examples of familial genetic genius, but he carefully selected his examples to include only such cases (Ishikawa 1930, 420).

He took a supportive stance toward eugenics' saying that attention should be paid to human heredity (Ishikawa 1928). But his later support for eugenics is clear:

Just as the male honeybee is slaughtered when it is determined to be harmful to the hive, we must remove all elements that are harmful to our national security and development (Ishikawa 1936, 420).

Along with Ishikawa, Oka Asajirō[2] contributed to the popularization of evolution and genetics, particularly by writing for the general public. He graduated from Tokyo Imperial University in 1891. Later, Oka was engaged in the research of invertebrate taxonomy as a professor of the Tokyo Higher Normal School.[3] His 1925 book *Shinkaron kōwa*[4] [Discourse on evolution theory] was published fourteen consecutive times. While Oka kept his distance from eugenics, he did participate as a founding member of the Japan Society of Race Hygiene.

Oka appears to have been a Lamarckist[5] who believed in the heredity of acquired characteristics. He pointed out the inconsistencies and the limitations of Mendel's genetics and evolution theory: " If genes are unchangeable, then evolution never occurred. ... The temperature affecting the body color of certain insects causes a change in its germ plasm as well" (Oka 1917, 288-290). He insisted that Mendel's laws could not explain the epigenetic[6] expression of genes nor macroevolution.[7] In his books, he continued to point out the limitations of Mendel's genetics behind eugenics:

I have no ideas opposing eugenics. ... However, I am worried that we will be disappointed if we expect that we will be able to completely improve people solely by eugenic measures. ... Our knowledge of genetics is still in a primitive stage. We've only just begun our encounter, and we do not know what direction the study of heredity will take in the future (Oka 1918, 533-534).

However, in an earlier 1905 article, Oka recommended eugenic policy based on

1. R. パール   2. 丘浅次郎   3. 東京高等師範学校   4. 進化論講話
5. ラマルキスト   6. エピジェネティクス（後成遺伝学）   7. 大進化

natural selection and social Darwinism:

> If we unnaturally protect inferior or harmful human beings and make possible their proliferation, progress in racial improvement cannot be expected. Straining to keep alive a weak-bodied person, who will leave behind the same kind of offspring to cause trouble for future generations may appear to be a fine task consistent with a spirit of benevolence. But, in fact, we are putting an unnecessary burden on people of coming ages, and they will be the victims of our present actions. Putting aside the empty theory of merely protecting human rights, we need to at least clamp down on leaving behind inferior descendants (Oka 1905, 572–573).

Another biologist that should not be overlooked is Yamanouchi Shigeo[1] (see Otsubo 2005 and 2013). After graduating from the Tokyo Higher Normal School, he entered Columbia University in 1904 and afterwards worked with John Coulter of Chicago University—the first professor to adopt eugenics into the curriculum. He learned genetics and eugenics from professors like Charles B. Davenport and carried out his cytogenetical research of seaweed. After returning to Japan in 1913, Yamanouchi began work as a professor at his alma mater and also worked closely with Naruse Jinzō,[2] president of the Japan Women's University, teaching genetics and eugenics. In addition to teaching, he participated in social movements. He was a founding member of the Japan Society of Eugenics (1924), a supporter of the Japan Eugenic Exercise/Movement Association[3] (1926), and a founding member of the Japan Society of Race Hygiene (1930). Yamanouchi's work centered on eugenics, but like Ishikawa and Oka, he insisted on the importance of environment along with heredity. When the Great Kanto Earthquake of 1923 destroyed his laboratory, Yamanouchi went to America to do research. He returned to Japan just before the outbreak of U.S.-Japan war in 1941. For reasons unknown, Yamanouchi's advocacy of eugenics after his return was not seen.

Like these three biologists, agronomist Toyama Kametarō[4] also insisted on the importance of eugenics. He noted that "what can be done through education, law, medicine, and hygiene to improve society would be limited to that generation. Eugenics is necessary to cull out the bad elements of society and make fundamental improvements." But at the same time, he kept some distance from human improvement studies based on a primitive stage of genetics: "Human improvement studies are based on precise genetics and thus we must not forget that it should be developed by demonstrating accurate facts" (Toyama 1911, 5, 91).

The above-mentioned representative biologists and agronomists were interested in

1. 山内繁雄　　2. 成瀬仁蔵　　3. 日本優生学運動協会　　4. 外山亀太郎

eugenics, enlightened students and the public about eugenics based on Mendel's genetics, and took part in eugenic groups organized by journalists and educators. But they also maintained the importance of environment in human development, pointed out the academic immaturity of eugenics, and insisted that developing genetics was essential for eugenics.

4. Genetics Education and the Birth of the Japan Genetics Society

The Ministry of Education established Tohoku Imperial University[1] in 1907, and the Sapporo Agricultural School that had been established in 1875 became the Tohoku Imperial University's College of Agriculture. Tanaka Yoshimaro[2] graduated from the College of Agriculture in 1909 and organized "The Mendel Group" for the study of genetics in 1912. The following year, he began a series of lectures on genetics—the first in Japan (Miyayama 1967, 382).

The first course of genetics[3] was begun in Tokyo Imperial University's Department of Botany in 1918, taught by Fujii Kenjirō, who had studied cytogenetics in Europe. It began as a course endowed by financiers, Nomura Tokushichi[4] and his brothers, with a donation of 50,000 yen in Kyushu Electric Light & Railroad Co.[5] bonds and 10,000 yen in cash.[*5] The application for setting up the course revealed an interest in eugenics: "In agriculture, horticulture, and animal husbandry, the improvement of all breeds opens a new path to racial improvement and becomes a matter of eugenics, a part of genetics" (Miyayama 1967, 382-383).

In 1915, prior to the establishment of the genetics course at Tokyo Imperial University, Abe Ayao[6] (Chiba Horticultural High School at Matsudo)[*6] founded the Japanese Society of Breeding[7] with Nohara Shigeroku[8] (Tokyo Imperial University), Toyama, Tanaka and three others. Publication of the society's journal *Nihon ikushu gakkai hō*[9] [Japanese Society of Breeding Reports] started in 1916. In the list of 196 members in the second issue were Nagai Hisomu[10] (Tokyo Imperial Unversity's Medical College) and Yamanouchi Shigeo

In June 1920, the Japanese Society of Breeding was reorganized to become the Genetics Society of Japan.[11] This society grew, expanding its membership to 634 by 1932. When compared to the Genetics Society in the U. K. (1921), it cannot be said that the founding of the Genetics Society of Japan was late.

1. 東北帝国大学　2. 田中義麿　3. 遺伝学講座　4. 野村徳七
5. 九州電灯鉄道株式会社　6. 安部文夫　7. 日本育種学会　8. 野原重六
9. 日本育種学会報　10. 永井潜　11. 日本遺伝学会

5. Geneticists and Eugenics

Three researchers, all of whom were at Tohoku Imperial University's College of Agriculture, were leaders in the spread of eugenics. Tanaka Yoshimaro studied sericulture and continued Toyama's research on silkworms after moving to Kyushu Imperial University. He published many articles and several books including the more than 1000-page *Genetics*[1] which was revised repeatedly from 1934–1965. Oguma Mamoru,[2] the first director of National Institute of Genetics in 1948, studied under entomologist Matsumura Shōnen.[3] To better grasp the development of genetics and eugenics in prewar Japan, a look at the contribution of these three is helpful.

Matsumura's name was among the founders of Ikeda's Eugenic Exercise/Movement Association. His book *Shinka to Shisō*[4] [Evolution and Ideology, 1925] shows that he was a radical social Darwinist, grounded in an unbending philosophy of natural selection and anti-Christian. Though he did not give a well-organized description of eugenics in this book, his stance reflects a strong affinity with eugenic thinking.

Tanaka was also a strong nationalist. In 1924 he made an appeal "for the important issue in today's Japan to improve the race in order to build a superior Yamato race[5]" (Tanaka 1924, 33). Subsequently in a 1925 article, Tanaka analyzed America's anti-Japanese immigration policy and insisted on the pressing need for improving the Yamato race and the establishment of a Eugenics Research Institute (Tanaka 1925, 45-46). Tanaka, along with Kawamura Tamiji[6] (Kyoto Imperial University Faculty of Science), Ōshima Hiroshi (Kyushu Imperial University Faculty of Agriculture), Miyake, and other geneticists were founding members of the Japan Society of Eugenics, the Eugenic Exercise/Movement Association, and the Japan Society of Race Hygiene. Tanaka was the most active genetics researcher who participated in the eugenic movement before and after the war.

In 1925 the Diet of Japan passed the *Chian Iji Hō*[7] [Peace Preservation Law], under which domestic freedom was suppressed. In the same year, a full-scale expansion of aggression into Asia began. Before university study, Tanaka had been a member of the Imperial Guard Division[8] and was a second lieutenant of Japanese army (Tanaka 1956, 49-51). The influence of such a career can be seen in his sympathy with nationalism and racism and his elation over victories in the wars with China and Russia, which enabled Japan to be counted among the world powers of that time. In Tanaka's 1939 presidential address to the annual meeting of the Genetics Society of Japan, he said:

If Japan is able to produce a prominent geneticist… , we will be able to demonstrate

---

1. 『遺伝学』（田中義麿）　2. 小熊捍　3. 松村松年　4. 『進化と思想』
5. 大和民族　6. 川村多實二　7. 治安維持法　8. 近衛師団

to the world the high level of Japanese culture and value of the Japanese race. ... How we can develop genetics? First, budgets should be increased, ... a course of genetics or eugenics should be set up in individual universities. Dr. Oguma's suggestion of the establishment of a national institute of genetics is appropriate for this time (Yuasa 1967, 344).

This speech exhibits his nationalism and patriotism and the role he thought scholarship played in the promotion of national prestige.

Oguma Mamoru also promoted the advancement of scholarship in a 1939 pamphlet he published himself, urging the establishment of a national genetics research institute[1] (Oguma 1939). It dealt with the topics of human resources, food production expansion, and the reinforcement of the Japanese race. He distributed this pamphlet to Diet members to persuade them of the institute's importance. When the national assembly convened in March 1940 and the National Eugenic Law[2] was discussed, Minister of Health and Welfare Yoshida Shigeru[3] replied that he would thoroughly consider the foundation of an institute. In August of the same year, the annual meeting of the Japan Genetics Society opened in Seoul, where a resolution to establish a National Institute of Genetics was adopted. In 1932 the government set up the Japan Society for the Promotion of Science[4] under the Ministry of Education in which a committee of eugenics was established by medical doctors and hygienists. In April 1941 another committee was set up, which dealt with genetics as basic science. Oguma served as chairman with Tanaka as project chief. This committee presented more than ten proposals to the Diet, none of which were actualized because of the onset of World War II.

Oguma's enthusiastic demand for a national institute of genetics reflects the atmosphere of Japan in the middle of the Sino-Japanese War. His petition was like a chimera made up of both belligerent, eugenic language praising war and scientific language giving a biological, genetic understanding of man. It began as follows:

A race is connected by blood.
The world is now facing a major shift in the situation of race as an axis. ... During these three years of holy war, Japan has finally tightened its bonds despite various anti-Japanese maneuvering and if it is to fully protect itself to the end in the struggle of the great task for a great Asia, it is a problem of blood (Oguma 1939).

A geneticist, whose opinions differed from these three, was Komai Taku[5] of Kyoto Imperial University.[6] He had studied under Thomas H. Morgan[7] at Columbia University

1. 国立遺伝研究所   2. 国民優生法   3. 吉田茂厚生大臣   4. 日本学術振興会
5. 駒井卓   6. 京都帝国大学   7. トーマス・H. モーガン

in 1927 and introduced hereditary research of the Drosophila fruit fly in Japan. He made efforts to spread knowledge of genetics and participated in various eugenics organizations with Tanaka and other geneticists. He had proposed the idea of an Institute of Genetics in 1930, earlier than Tanaka or Oguma (Komai 1930, 315-322). In 1944 he began by pointing out weaknesses in eugenics and then built up to full scale criticism (Komai 1944, 322-350):

> An anachronism occurred in that applied eugenics grew up before the genetics upon which it is based. ... Among those who are enthusiastic supporters of eugenics study and the eugenics system, most are laymen in genetics or partial laymen. ... Compared to the dramatic growth of genetics, eugenics did not advance at all (Komai 1944, 325).

In his 1934 book *Nihonjin no iden*[1] [Heredity of Japanese] and in many articles in eugenics journals, his comments always held fast to genetics. Around 1939, he voiced strong criticism of the National Eugenic Law. In a lecture at Kyoto Imperial University, he asserted:

> Galton, the proponent of eugenics, did not know genetics. The guiding principle of eugenics has remained at an earlier stage than Mendel's. When eugenicists observe complex hereditary phenomena, they come up with ridiculous and fallacious arguments (Ōshima 1988, 431).

Whether Komai used eugenics as an avenue for pursuing genetic study or whether his criticism of eugenics came as a result of his study in human genetics is unclear. But it is clear that Komai begin to distance himself from the eugenic movement by the end of World War II. Taking such a stand under the rigid rule of wartime nationalism and fascism undoubtedly required a good amount of determination and courage.

6. Foundation of the National Institute of Genetics

In November 1945 after the end of World War II, Oguma wrote a letter to the Ministry of Education, urging the immediate establishment of an institute of genetics. In 1946 the Genetics Society of Japan set up a preparatory committee for founding the institute and presented a formal petition to the Ministry of Education, which included the proposal to locate the institute on the site of the factory of the former Nakajima Aircraft

---

1. 『日本人の遺伝』

Company in Mishima, Shizuoka Prefecture.[1] The petition was approved in April 1947 and the Institute of Genetics Foundation[2] was tentatively established in May with an initial budget of 700,000 yen, of which 200,000 yen was donated by Central Equine Affairs Society[3] (Miyayama 1948a, 1948b).

The budget for the National Institute of Genetics passed the Ministry of Education's budget council in September 1947, and the petition for the installation of a laboratory was taken up in the First Diet session[4] after the adoption of the new constitution. The total planned three year budget of 200 million yen was initially approved by both Houses, but, new additions to the budget were rejected. Under the occupation of U. S. forces, all political and academic affairs were required to have permission of the General Headquarters (GHQ).[5] The Economic and Scientific Section[6] (ESS) of the GHQ inspected the planned site and made a detailed report of the foundation.

In July 1948, the draft budget of ¥3,356,000 for the first fiscal year was approved by the Diet. Putting aside the question of expense, the National Institute of Genetics[7] was established on June 1, 1949. It had taken ten years in between wars, but at long last, the efforts of Oguma, Tanaka, and others bore fruit. Oguma became the first president and director of the cytogenetics laboratory, Tanaka director of the genetic morphology laboratory, and Komai director of physiological genetic laboratory. The institute began with three laboratories and nineteen researchers. There was no "laboratory of racial heredity" that had appeared in Oguma's pre-war plan, and words related to eugenics or racial hygiene were not to be found. In addition, this institution was organized as a purely basic biological research organization, separated from other administrative organizations, just as Oguma had described in it 1944.

7. Postwar Promotion of Eugenics in the Magazine *Iden*

In addition to their academic bulletin *The Japanese Journal of Genetics*[8] (established in 1921), the Genetics Society of Japan began a publication for the promotion of genetics titled *Iden*[9] [Heredity] in November 1947. In the first issue, one of the editing committee members, Masui Kiyoshi[10] (Department of Agriculture, Tokyo University), described its purpose as being to develop improved varieties as a part of a national food policy and to improve the genetic quality of Japanese race for the postwar rehabilitation of Japan (Masui 1947, 1-2). Tanaka wrote a subsequent article, emphasizing the implementation of eugenics just as he had before the war,

We need to root out weeds as soon as possible. ... The first thing that must be done

1. 静岡県三島   2. 財団法人遺伝研究所   3. 中央馬事会   4. 第1回国会
5. 連合国最高司令官総司令部   6. 経済科学局   7. 国立遺伝研究所
8. 『遺伝学雑誌』   9. 『遺伝』   10. 増井清

for the reconstruction of a civilized nation is to do a eugenics study and to build its shape. Thus a new Japan in the name of eugenic Japan[1] would first appear on the stage of the new century. ... Firstly, if a large number of hereditary criminals,[2] persons with low mental abilities, or mentally ill persons are mixed in with our seventy million compatriots and their ratio continues to increase year by year, what will happen? Even at present our citizens are bearing an almost too heavy burden, but if they have to bear the additional burden of the genetically defective, it will only delay the rebuilding of our homeland. ... It is important that we not wait until it is too late to deal with the interracial marriages[3] which are becoming a problem in recent days (Tanaka 1947, 3-5).

His last comments suggest that he feared Japanese blood would be mixed with that of Koreans who were brought to Japan as forced laborers during the war or with that of the American servicemen of the occupation forces.

During the process of forming the Eugenic Protection Law,[4] an article about forced sterilization[5] and human rights[6] presented the opinions of eleven academics. Eight thought that compulsory sterilization was legal or at least unavoidable for the public interest—an opinion shared by Tanaka:

Because serious hereditary defects affect not only person in question, but these defects are also passed on to the descendants, their bad influence on society is much more serious than those of people with infectious diseases or violent persons. The necessity of forced sterilization is only natural for ethnic cleansing[7] (*Iden* 4 [1950], 10-11).

Komai wrote a dissenting opinion, contrasting that of Tanaka. He noted that the most enthusiastic supporters of sterilization were not those with genetic training. He agreed that sterilization would reduce the burden on care givers, but insisted that limits needed to be set by experts, not those with a limited understanding of heredity. (*Iden* 4 [1950], 10-11).

After the war, Japanese society faced the challenges of rebuilding[8] from the ashes of bombed and burned cities and dealing with a sudden increase in population due to the return of repatriated soldiers. As a result, threatening population problems surfaced on a scale larger than before the war. In 1948, the National Eugenic Law, which had been in effect since 1940, was revised, and a new Eugenic Protection Law was established. This new law aimed to legalize induced abortion for eugenic reasons, but in 1950 it was

1. 優生日本　2. 遺伝的犯罪　3. 人種間結婚　4. 優生保護法　5. 強制断種
6. 人権　7. 民族浄化　8. 戦後復興

revised again to allow abortion for economic reasons. Such a social situation can be seen as a reason for the push to establish the National Institute of Genetics, despite the postwar national crisis. In addition, the influence of geneticists, who wrote many articles on eugenics in *Iden*, can be seen in the enactment of both laws.

At the annual meeting of Genetics Society of Japan in October 1947, just before the first publication of *Iden*, Lysenko's genetic theory[1*7] was introduced, resulting in opposing opinions among the members. As supporters of Mendel's and Morgan's theories, Komai, Tanaka, and Shinotō Yoshito[2] were among those who were critical. In October 1948, a round-table talk was included in *Iden* (2, 14-20, 22-25). This criticism of Lysenkoism by Japanese scientists also brought a new awareness of the importance of keeping science independent of political authority. Genetics, began to distance itself from politics. Thereafter, a propaganda-like presentation of eugenics gradually disappeared from *Iden* articles.

From that time on, sporadic articles appeared which discussed eugenics based on population genetics of the adverse selection of human civilization and the accumulation of genes not beneficial to survival. In 1965 the Genetics Society of Japan held a symposium "*Idengaku kara mita jinrui no shōrai*" [The future of mankind as seen from genetics] to commemorate the 100th anniversary of Mendel's discovery. Kimura Motoo,[3] researcher at the National Institute of Genetics and known world-wide for his "theory of neutral genes,"[4] gave a lecture about the evolutionary direction of mankind and genetic betterment, in which he pointed out that adverse selection due to a decline in infant mortality and a low birthrate was inescapable. This idea of the necessity of eugenic measures is seen clearly in his 1988 book:

> As a living organism, a person is rooted in the existence of various human beings, whose form is translated from the genetic commands found in the nucleus of the fertilized egg. Based on this, when the commands permit degeneration, the final result is the degeneration of mankind. It may be a matter of tens of thousands of years, but mankind must use the majority of its knowledge, efforts, and material resources for more constructive, more expansive undertakings, rather than for measures dealing with observable characteristics. To do this, eugenic measures are absolutely necessary (Kimura 1988, 271-272).

His recommendations also included screening and removing defective genes in the early stages of development before birth.

1. ルイセンコ学説   2. 篠遠喜人   3. 木村資生   4. 中立遺伝子説

Concluding Remarks

Even though genome science has made remarkable progress, many unsolved problems remain. Such problems include clarification of the non-coded region[1] that occupies 95% of the human genome,[2] the epigenetic control of gene expression by the environment, and the gene expression control network.[3] Unraveling one problem only raises new ones. The present state of contemporary genetics is that we are still far from having a clear picture of evolutionary factors. Therefore, caution should be exercised when advocating the deletion of defective genes since the mechanisms of gene regulation and gene evolution have not yet been made clear. We need to make a fresh start from the eugenics of the early twentieth century.

On the other hand, mankind's ability to produce goods has increased incredibly, and the social structure of human society has changed drastically during the last 100 years. It is no exaggeration to say that the reasons for the existence of eugenics—adverse selection and the pressure of evolutionary selection—have changed considerably. By changing our strategy, a dramatic increase in the production of goods can lead to a new era, one in which, rather than seeking a few geniuses, we increase the amount of information in society, devise ways of improving the developmental environment for individuals, and collectively pursue the possibilities of mankind. Relief from physical labor reduces the impact of adverse selection which might have drastically reduced the number of disabled persons, and the boundary between disabled persons and able-bodied persons becomes ambiguous. So the effects of adverse selection cannot be as easily argued as was done in the past. Furthermore, a society that accepts minorities like women and disabled persons is certain to give rise to new moral models and values and a greater height of quality. It is clear that the increase of minorities does not produce a burden on society. The stability and evolutionary mechanism of the human gene group which Kimura pursued is an important problem for population genetics to solve. But this solution needs to be worked out on a completely different playing field than that of nineteenth century eugenics and needs to be based on new knowledge.

Notes

*1 After studying abroad at the laboratory of August Weismann at the University of Freiburg in 1886, Ishikawa also published a translation of Weismann's "*Über den Rückschritt in der Natur*," entitled "*Banbutsu taika shinsetsu*" [A new theory of the degeneration of organisms] in 1889.

*2 The oldest description of the evolutionary theory may be *Kitagō dan*[4] (Story of the Northern

---

1. DNA 非コード領域　　2. ヒトゲノム　　3. 遺伝子発現制御ネットワーク
4. 『北郷談』

*3　This translation is from Jennifer Robertson (2002, 12). *Undō* can be translated both as exercise and movement.

*4　The reference here is to Raymond Pearl, a biologist at Johns Hopkins University in Baltimore, Maryland. In 1927, he published an article in *The American Mercury* magazine entitled "Biology of Superiority" (12:257–266). This first biological critique of eugenics and of Galton made national headlines in American newspapers.

*5　This financial support appears to follow the example of the Carnegie Foundation's funding of the Institute of Experimental Evolution in 1904 and Mrs. E. H. Harriman's funding of the Eugenic Records Office at Cold Spring Harbor in 1910.

*6　In 1919 Abe became the principal of the agriculture and forestry technical school attached to the Taiwanese governor-general's office. He graduated from the faculty of literature but studied selective breeding of plants as a geneticist and was an active eugenicist.

*7　Soviet agronomist Trofim D. Lysenko (1898–1976) asserted that it is possible to inherit environmentally acquired characteristics, reflecting Neo-Lamarckism and anti-Mendelism. He also used governmental authority to repress his critics. His theory was discredited around 1950.

References

Ameda Ei'ichi ［雨田英一］. 2000. "Fukuzawa Yukichi no 'Maruhadaka no kyōsō' to 'Jinshu kairyō' no shisō" ［福沢諭吉の「丸裸の競走」と「人種改良」の思想 Fukuzawa Yukichi's Ideas on "stark-naked competition" and "race betterment"］ in *Tōyōbunkakenkyū* ［東洋文化研究 *J. Asian Cultures*］ 2 (Mar.), 385–418.

Araya Buei ［新谷武衛］. 1950. "Nihon gakujutsu shinkōkai to idengaku (1)" ［日本学術振興会と遺伝学(1) The Japan Society for the Promotion of Science and Genetics (1)］ in *Iden* ［遺伝 *Heredity*］ 4, 460–462.

Bartholomew, James R. 1989. *The Formation of Science in Japan*. New Haven: Yale University.

Darbishire, Arthur D. 1902. "Note on the Results of Crossing Japanese Waltzing Mice with European Albino Races" in *Biometrika* 2:1, 101–113. (Japanese translation by Kuwano Hisataka ［桑野久任］. 1903. *Dōbutsugaku zasshi* ［動物学雑誌 *Zoological magazine*］ 15, 210–216.)

Darwin, Charles. 1859. *On the Origin of Species by Means of Natural Selection, or the Preservation of Favoured Races in the Struggle for Life*. London: John Murray. (Japanese translation by Tachibana Senzaburō ［立花銑三郎］ 1896. *Seibutsushigen ichimei shugenron* ［生物始原一名種源論 The origin of living things or the origin of species］ Tokyo: Keizai Zasshisha.)

—— 1871. *Human Descent and Selection in Relation to Sex*. London: John Murray. (Japanese

---

1.　葵川信近

translation by Kōdzu Senzaburō［神津専三郎］1881. *Jinsoron*［人祖論 Human Descent］. Tokyo: Yamanaka Hyōbei.)

Fukuzawa Yukichi［福澤諭吉］. 1881. *Jijishōgen*［時事小言 Short essay of current news］. Tokyo: Yamanaka Ichibei and Maruzen Shosha.

Galton, Francis. 1869. *Hereditary Genius*. London: Macmillan. (Japanese translation by Haraguchi Tsuruko［原口鶴子］1916. *Tensai to Iden*［天才と遺伝 Genius and Heredity］. Tokyo: Waseda Daigaku Shuppankai.)

Hilgendorf, Franz M. 1878. *Seibutsu shinron dai ippen*［生物新論　第 1 編 New theory of biology Part 1］. Matsubara Shin'nosuke［松原新之介］, trans. Tokyo: Bansuisha.

Huxley, Thomas H. 1863. On the origin of species: or the causes of the phenomena of organic nature. A course of six lectures to working men. New York: D. Appleton. (Japanese translation by Izawa Shūji［伊澤修二］. 1879. *Seishu genshiron*［生種原始論］. Tokyo: Mori Shigetō. 1889. *Shinka genron*［進化原論 Principles of evolution］. Tokyo: Maruzen.)

Iden Editorial Committee ［遺伝編集委員会］. 1950. "Hagaki kaitō: Kyōseidanshu to jinken mondai"［葉書回答：強制断種と人権問題 Answers by post card: Forced sterilization and human rights］in *Iden* ［遺伝 Heredity］4, 10-11.

Ikeda Shigenori［池田淋義］. 1926. *Yūseigakuteki shakaikaizō undō*［優生学的社会改造運動 Eugenics and social remodeling movement］. Tokyo: Gakujutsu Koen Tsushinsha.

Ikeno Sei'ichirō ［池野誠一郎］. 1906. *Shokubutsu keitōgaku* ［植物系統学 Phylogenetic botany］. Tokyo: Shōkabō.

Inatomi Eijirō ［稲富栄治郎］. 1956. *Meiji shoki no kyōikushisō no kenkyū*［明治初期の教育思想の研究 The study of educational ideology in early Meiji period］. Tokyo: Fukumura Shoten.

Ishikawa Chiyomatsu［石川千代松］. 1928. *Ningen*［人間 Human being］. Tokyo: Banrikakushobo.

——. 1930. *Ningen to shinka*［人間と進化 Humans and evolution］. Tokyo: Kobunsha.

——. 1936. "Dōbutsu no shinka to kokka"［動物の進化と国家　The evolution of animals and the state］in *Toyō Gakugei Zasshi*,［東洋学芸雑誌 Journal of Oriental Art］33:9, 420.

Kihara Hitoshi［木原均］, et al., ed. 1972. *Reimeiki nihon no seibutsugakushi*［黎明期日本の生物学史 The history of biological sciences in old Japan］, 337-382. Tokyo: Yokendo.

—— et al., ed. 1988. *Kindai nihon seibutsugakusha shōden*［近代日本生物学者小伝 Short biographies of modern Japanese biologists］. Tokyo: Hirakawa Shuppansha.

Kimura Motoo［木村資生］. 1988. *Seibutsu shinka wo kangaeru*［生物進化を考える Thinking about the evolution of organisms］. Tokyo: Iwanami Shoten.

Komai Taku［駒井卓］. 1934. *Nihonjin no iden*［日本人の遺伝 Heredity of Japanese］. Tokyo: Yokendo.

——. 1930. *Seibutsugaku sōwa*［生物学叢話 Collection of biology anecdotes］. Tokyo: Kaizosha.

―――. 1944. *Idengaku sōwa* [遺伝学叢話 Collection of genetics anecdotes]. Kyoto: Torikabutoshorin.

Masui Kiyoshi [増井清]. 1947. "*Iden* no kankō ni atatte" [「遺伝」の刊行に当たって On the publication of *Iden*] in *Iden* [遺伝 *Heredity*] 1:1, 1-2.

Matsubara Yōko [松原洋子]. 2000. "Mendel idengaku no jyuyō" [メンデル遺伝学の受容 Reception of Mendel's Genetics] in *Seibutsugakushi kenkyū* [生物学史研究 *Japanese Journal of the History of Biology*] 66, 89-91.

Matsumura Shōnen [松村松年]. 1925. *Shinka to shisō* [進化と思想 Evolution and thought]. Tokyo: Dainippon Yubenkai.

Miyayama Heihachirō [宮山平八郎]. 1948a. "Kokuritsu idengaku kenkyūsho setsuritsu ni itaru made (1)" [国立遺伝学研究所設立に至るまで(1) Until the establishment of the national genetics research institute (1)] in *Iden* [遺伝 *Heredity*] 2, 324-325

―――. 1948b. "Kokuritsu idengaku kenkyūsho setsuritsu ni itaru made (2)" [国立遺伝学研究所設立に至るまで(2) Until the establishment of the national genetics research institute (2)] in *Iden* [遺伝 *Heredity*] 2, 422-424

―――. 1967. "Daigaku no idengaku kōza" [大学の遺伝学講座 University course of genetics] in *Idengaku no ayumi: Menderu idenhōsoku 100 nenkinen* [遺伝学のあゆみ：メンデル遺伝法則100年記念 The path of genetics: Centennial anniversary of Mendel's laws], Mendel centennial anniversary publication committee, ed., 379-385. Tokyo: Shokabo.

Miyoshi Manabu [三好学]. 1905. *Shinpen shokubutsugaku kōgi gekan* [新編植物学講義 下巻 New lectures of botany, volume 2]. Tokyo: Fuzanbo.

Morse, Edward S. 1883. *Dōbutsu shinkaron* [動物進化論 Theory of animal evolution], Ishikawa Chiyomatsu [石川千代松], trans. Tokyo: Higashio Kamejirō.

―――. 1990 [1917]. *Japan Day by Day*. Atlanta: Cheroky Publishing Company.

Oguma Mamoru [小熊捍]. 1939. *Kokuritsu idenkenkyūsho setsuritsu no kyūmu* [国立遺伝研究所設立の急務 The urgent task of establishing a national institute of genetics]. Sapporo: Oguma Mamoru.

Oka Asajirō [丘浅次郎]. 1905. "Shinka to eisei" [進化と衛生 Evolution and hygiene] in *Kokka igakukai zasshi* [国家医学会雑誌 *National Association Medical of Sciences Magazine*] 221, 567-575.

―――. 1917. "Iden no chūshinmondai" [遺伝の中心問題 The main problem of heredity] in *Shinrigaku kenkyū* [心理学研究 *Psychological Research*] 12:69, 34-40.

―――. 1918. *Saishin idenron* [最新遺伝論 The latest theory of heredity]. Tokyo: Rokumeikan.

―――. 1925. *Shinkaron kōwa* [進化論講話 Discourse on evolution theory]. Tokyo: Tokyo Kaiseikan.

Onaga, Lisa. 2010. "Toyama Kametarō and Vernon Kellogg: silkworm inheritance experiments in Japan, Siam and the United States, 1900-1912" in *Journal of the History of Biology* 43:2

(Summer), 215-64.

Ōshima Chōzō ［大島長造］. 1988. "Komai Taku—bunrigaku, keitōgaku kara idengaku he" ［駒井卓―分類学，系統学から遺伝学へ Komai Taku—from taxonomy and phylogeny to genetics］, 427-434. (See Kihara 1988.)

Ōshima Hiroshi ［大島廣］. 1909. "Iden ni tsuite" ［遺伝に就いて On heredity］ in *The Zoological Magazine*, 21, 24-29.

Otsubo, Sumiko. 2005. "Between Two Worlds: Yamanouchi Shigeo and Eugenics in Early Twentieth-Century Japan" in *Annals of Science* 62:2, 205-31.

――― ［大坪寿美子］. 2013. "Nichibei yūseigaku no setten shokubutsugakusha Yamanouchi Shigeo wo chūshin ni shite" ［日米優生学の接点　植物学者山内繁雄を中心にして A point of contact between Japan and US: Botanist Yamanouchi Shigeo］" in *Seimei no Rinri* 3 ［生命の倫理 3　Ethics of life 3］, Yamazaki Kiyoko ［山崎喜代子］, ed., 131-160. Fukuoka: Kyushu Daigaku Shuppankai.

Shibata Keita ［柴田桂太］. 1904. "Rōzenberuhi shi 'Mousen goke ni okeru gensūbunretsu ni tsuite'" ［ローゼンベルヒ氏『もうせんごけに於ける減数分裂に就いて』 Mr. Rosenberg "About meiosis in Dosera"］ in *Shokubutsugaku zasshi* ［植物学雑誌 Botany Magazine］ 18, 126-127.

Spencer, Herbert. 1880. *Shishi kyōikuron* ［斯氏教育論 Spencer's education theory］, Seki Shinpachi ［尺振八］, trans. Tokyo: Ministry of Education.

Tanaka Yoshimaro ［田中義麿］. 1924. "Ningen honshitsu no kaizen ga kyūmu" ［人間本質の改善が急務 Betterment of mankind's essential qualities is urgent］ in *Igaku oyobi ningen* ［医学及び人間 Medical Science and mankind］ 2:3, 33.

―――. 1925. "Yūseigaku kara mita hainichimondai ［優生学から観た排日問題 Anti-Japanese problem as seen from eugenics］ in *Yūseigaku* ［優生学 Eugenics］ 2, 39-46.

―――. 1937. *Iden gaku* ［遺伝学 Genetics］. Tokyo: Shokabo.

―――. 1947. "Idengaku kenkyū no hitsuyō" ［遺伝学研究の必要 The necessity of genetics research］ in *Iden* ［遺伝 Heredity］ 1, 3-4.

Toyama Kametarō ［外山亀太郎］. 1906. "Kasan no zasshu ni tsuite" ［家蚕の雑種について Hybrids of silkworms］ in *Tokyo teikoku daigaku nōkadaigaku gakujutsu hōkoku* ［東京帝国大学農科大学学術報告　Bulletin of the College of Agriculture Tokyo Imperial University］ 7, 259-393.

―――. 1909. *Yōsanron* ［養蚕論 Sericulture theory］. Tokyo: Maruyamasha.

―――. 1910. "Idengaku no shinpo to jinsei no kankei" ［遺伝学の進歩と人生の関係 Progress of genetics and relationship to life］ in *Rigakkai* ［理学界 Science world］ 8, 1-6.

―――. 1911. *Jinruikairyōgaku to seibutsukairyōgaku* ［人類改良学と生物改良学 The study of the improvement of mankind and the study of the improvement of animals］ in *Shin Nippon* ［新日本 New Japan］ 1, 89-92.

Ueno Masuzō [上野益三]. 1988a. "Edowādo Shiruvesutā Mōsu—Nihon saisho no dōbutsugaku kyōjyu" [エドワード・シルヴェスター・モース—日本最初の動物学教授 Edward Sylvester Morse—Japan's first zoology professor], 77-85. (See Kihara 1988.)

———. 1988b. "Yatabe Ryōkichi —Nihon hatsu no shokubutsugaku kyōjyu" [矢田部良吉—日本初の植物学教授 Yatabe Ryōkichi—The first Japanese professor of botany], 86-93. (See Kihara 1988.)

Weismann, August. 1886. *Über den Rückschritt in der Natur.* Freiburg i.B.: J.C.B. Mohr. (Japanese translation by Ishikawa Chiyomatsu [石川千代松], *Banbutsu taika shinsetsu* [万物退化新説 A new theory of the degeneration of organisms]. Tokyo: Ogawado.)

Yuasa Akira [湯浅明]. 1967. "Gakkai" [学会 Academic societies] in *Idengaku no ayumi: Menderu idenhōsoku 100 nen kinen* [遺伝学のあゆみ: メンデル遺伝法則 100 年記念 The path of genetics: Centennial anniversary of Mendel's laws], Mendel centennial anniversary publication committee, ed., 341-378. Tokyo: Shokabo.

Xu, Yan. [許艶]. 1991. "Katō Hiroyuki ni okeru shinkaron no jyuyō to tenkai: 'nōryokushugi' kyōikushisō no seisei" [加藤弘之における進化論の受容と展開:「能力主義」教育思想の生成] The acceptance of evolutionism by Hiroyuki Kato—The formation of 'meritocracy' in Japanese educational thought] in *Bulletin of the Faculty of Education, University of Tokyo* 31, 85-93.

Chapter 2   *Eugenics and Psychiatric Medicine*

Kitagaki Tōru

  Before discussing the relationship of psychiatry in modern Japan to eugenics, it is necessary to take a glance at the relationship that this field of medicine had in general to society in those days. Roughly speaking, such a relationship can be traced partly with the term "*seishin eisei*"[1] [mental hygiene]. The word "hygiene" has its origin from the Greek word that means "health," while the Japanese characters "*ei-sei*" literally signify "the protection of life." Therefore, one can consider "*seishin eisei*" or mental hygiene primarily as the medical practice which is carried out in order to protect people's life from mental disease and illness. But this term can also be considered as a police measure, which protects normal people from the mentally ill or mentally disordered. Psychiatrists have thus had a double function in society, that is, the medical treatment and care of patients on the one hand, and the protection of society from these patients by isolating them elsewhere, on the other. With a brief historical review of early twentieth century Japan, we will first examine this Janus-faced figure of psychiatry.

1. Psychiatric Medicine as a Tool of Social Protection

  Seishinbyōsha kangohō[2] [The Mental Patients' Custody Act], established in 1900, was one which endeavored to standardize practices on a national level. Up until this time each prefecture had conducted these practices for the mentally ill on a local level. This law stipulated procedures for the confinement of a patient, either in a mental hospital or at a private home, while designating a custodian who was responsible for the treatment. (When a proper custodian could not be found, it would be the local administrative head of the patient's place of residence who assumed this status.) Yet since there were very few public mental hospitals in those days, most of the patients were obliged to be confined in their own home. According to this law, the police would intervene in the procedures of confinement, which required the permission of the administrative authority. In this way, the Mental Patients' Custody Act seemed to be established, not for medical treatment of

---

1. 精神衛生   2. 精神病者監護法

the mentally ill, but for social protection which aimed to separate patients from the rest of the people. (In Tokyo, the administrator responsible for this law was the chief of the metropolitan police, not the governor of Tokyo.) It was quite late, in 1938, that the Ministry of Health and Welfare[1] was created, and until that time, hygiene administration was conducted by the Central Hygiene Bureau of the Home Ministry,[2] and the lowest level of this administration was carried out by police stations in each district. So the home custody[3] of a patient obliged the family to act partly as an agent of the police, by confining a member of the family in their own home and separating him or her from society. Besides, whether at home or in a mental hospital, the cost of confinement had to be paid by the confined or the custodian. Such a system of home custody continued to exist for half a century, until 1950, when the *Seishineiseihō*[4] [Mental Hygiene Act] was established after the defeat of Japan in the Pacific War. According to Okada Yasuo,[5] one of the leading historians of Japanese psychiatry, this system of home custody formed an archetype of mental treatment in Japan, and its principal features remain even nowadays as an undercurrent (Okada 2002a, 141).

As already noted, the number of mental hospitals, whether public or private, was extremely limited when the Mental Patients' Custody Act was introduced in 1900. It was the Kyoto Insane Asylum,[6] built in 1875 by Kyoto prefecture, which was the first public mental hospital to be established in the Meiji period as Japan was modernizing. This hospital, located on the premises of Nanzenji Temple,[7] was soon abolished in 1882, due to financial reasons (although it continued to exist as a private clinic). In 1879, Tokyo Insane Asylum[8] was the second public mental hospital to be established. It was originally situated in Ueno, but moved to Mukōgaoka, and then to Sugamo (Sugamo Hospital of Tokyo Prefecture). When it was moved again to Setagaya, in the western suburb of the capital, it was renamed Matsuzawa Hospital of Tokyo Prefecture.[9] On the other hand, since the 1870s, some specialized wards for mental disease patients began to be set up in Army Hospitals[10] nationwide. As for private hospitals, they were built mainly in larger cities, such as Tokyo and Osaka. The number of beds in all of these hospitals was far below those required by the Mental Patients' Custody Act, but continued to increase steadily.

In 1919, the Imperial Parliament adopted the *Seishinbyōinhō*[11] [Mental Hospital Act], which enabled the Home Minister to order the prefectural governor to set up mental hospitals. This law provided that the cost of constructing the hospital would be partially paid for by the central government. And, in contrast to the Mental Patients' Custody Act, it also stipulated that the chief of the mental hospital would assume responsibility for confinement of the patient. The Mental Hospital Act thus declared a policy of public

1. 厚生省　2. 内務省衛生局　3. 私宅監置　4. 精神衛生法　5. 岡田靖雄
6. 京都癲狂院　7. 南禅寺　8. 東京府癲狂院　9. 東京府立松沢病院
10. 衛戍病院　11. 精神病院法

responsibility for psychiatric treatment, transferring the agent of confinement from the family to medical doctors. But in reality, this law did not enable the construction of mental hospitals promptly enough to satisfy the demand. The project of constructing national hospitals was discussed, but failed to be realized. Until Japan's defeat in the Pacific War, mental public hospitals built on the basis of this law were as follows: Matsuzawa Hospital of Tokyo Prefecture (already built in 1879 but officially authorized under this law in 1920), Nakanomiya Hospital of Osaka Prefecture[1] (established in 1926), Sekō-in of Kanagawa Prefecture[2] (established in 1929), Chikushi Sanitarium of Fukuoka Prefecture[3] (established in 1931), the Sanitarium of Kagoshima Prefecture[4] (first built as a psychiatric ward of the Kagoshima Public Hospital in 1924, and recognized as an independent institution in 1931), the Mental Hospital of Aichi prefecture[5] (established 1932), Kōfū-ryō of Hyōgo Prefecture[6] (established in 1937), and the Mental Hospital of Kyoto Prefecture[7] (established in 1945).

Leading psychiatrists of the time, like Kure Shūzō,[8] Tokyo Imperial University professor of psychiatry, and Miyake Kōichi,[9] his successor, participated in the enactment of the Mental Hospital Act. After studying in Germany and Austria, Kure came back to Japan in 1901 and was appointed professor of the Medical School of Tokyo Imperial University, as well as chief of Sugamo Hospital of Tokyo Prefecture.[10] In this hospital, he tried to introduce humanitarian treatment of patients, abolishing the restraint[11] system used up to that time. When Sugamo Hospital was moved and renamed Matsuzawa Hospital, the director was Kure and the vice director was Miyake. The head doctor was Shimoda Mitsuzō,[12] and on the staff of doctors was Kaneko Junji.[13] Just as Miyake succeeded Kure at the Imperial University of Tokyo, he also became the Director of Matsuzawa Hospital. Kure, who opposed the use of instruments of restraint in the hospital was also critical of the treatment of patients in the home custody system. In order to survey the actual situation of the mentally ill in home confinement, his assistants were sent out, from 1910 to 1916, to visit 361 patients in fifteen prefectures. This survey resulted in a report titled *Seishinbyōsha shitakukanchi no jikkyō oyobi sono tōkeiteki kansatsu*[14] [Description and Statistical observation of the mentally ill under home custody], published in 1918, and co-authored by Kure and Kashida Gorō[15] (Kure, Kashida 2012).

Concerning the administration of mental hygiene, a Central Hygiene Committee[16] was created in 1879 as a consultative body (the president was Mori Arinori[17]), and a local commission was set up in each prefecture. But the role of the central hygiene committee, whose members numbered only thirteen, was quite limited at the beginning. It was not until World War I that the hygienic administration developed actively, changing its role

1. 大阪府立中宮病院   2. 神奈川県立芹香院   3. 福岡県立筑紫保養院
4. 鹿児島県立保養院   5. 愛知県立精神病院   6. 兵庫県立光風寮
7. 京都府立精神病院   8. 呉秀三   9. 三宅鑛一   10. 東京府立巣鴨病院   11. 拘束
12. 下田光造   13. 金子準二   14. 『精神病者私宅監置ノ実況及ビ其統計的観察』
15. 樫田五郎   16. 内務省中央衛生会   17. 森有礼

from preventive to promotional policy, which aimed to directly advance the health of the whole nation. In 1916, the Research Committee for Health[1] was established with 34 members, among whom we find the names Nagai Hisomu,[2] Fujikawa Yū,[3] and Takano Iwasaburō.[4] This Committee had eight sections of research: i) babies, children, adolescents, ii) tuberculosis,[5] iii) sexually transmitted disease, iv) leprosy,[6] v) mental disease, vi) food, clothing, and shelter, vii) hygiene in rural areas (later including urban areas), viii) statistics. The fifth section specializing in mental disease had as its members Yanagisawa Yasutoshi,[7] Miyake Kōichi, Kurimoto Yoshikatsu,[8] Yokote Chiyonosuke,[9] and Noda Tadahiro.[10] One of the researches conducted by these members was concerning the number of patients who were either in a mental hospital or in home custody. (Those who actually conducted this research on the field were policemen.) The result showed a total of 64,934 patients in the nation (40,848 men and 24,086 women). This number greatly exceeded the one published by the Home Ministry, because it included "suspected cases" (Okada 2002a, 173).

When studying in Germany and Austria, Kure became aware of the existence of the "*Hilfsverein*" (association for the help of patients) in each mental hospital. After returning to Japan, he gave a lecture on this institution for the Japan Women's Association for Hygiene.[11] In this context, the Charity Association for the Help of Mental Patients[12] was established by the principal initiative of Kure's wife Minako.[13] The members were mainly the wives of medical school professors and famous doctors, while their husbands became associate members. The first president was Ōkuma Ayako[14] (wife of Ōkuma Shigenobu[15]), and the second Matsui Shōko[16] (sister of adopted child of Ōkuma). The first bulletin of this association was published in 1903, under the title *Shinshitsusha no kyūgo*[17] [Help for mental patients]. In 1924, this association opened a temporary help station on the grounds of Matsuzawa Hospital, in order to care for victims of the Great Earthquake. In 1927, it was renamed *Kyūchi-kai*[18] [Help Association], and adopted a system of directors in abolishing the distinction between regular members and associate members. The first director was Kure, and after his resignation, Miyake succeeded him. In 1929, the title of the bulletin was changed to *Kyūchikai kaihō*[19] [Bulletin of the Help Association], and sixty issues were published, the last one in 1941. In 1943, this association was incorporated, with the Japan Association of Mental Hospitals[20] and the Japan Association of Mental Hygiene,[21] into *Seishin Kōseikai*[22] [Association of Mental Welfare].

Just after the enforcement of the Mental Hospital Act, an organization was created in 1920 by psychiatric doctors. The first president was Kure, always like other cases, and after his death in 1932, it was Miyake who succeeded him. This organization was

1. 保健衛生調査会　2. 永井潜　3. 富士川游　4. 高野岩三郎　5. 結核
6. らい（ハンセン病）　7. 柳澤保恵　8. 栗本庸勝　9. 横手千代之助
10. 野田忠廣　11. 日本婦人衛生会　12. 精神病者慈善救治会　13. 呉岢子
14. 大隈綾子　15. 大隈重信　16. 松井正子　17. 『心疾者の救護』　18. 救治会
19. 『救治会々報』　20. 日本精神病院協会　21. 日本精神衛生協会　22. 精神厚生会

dissolved in 1935, and its property was divided in halves and donated to the Japan Association of Mental Hospitals and the Japan Association of Mental Hygiene. The Japan Association of Mental Hospitals originated from the council of presidents of public and substitute mental hospitals, held for the first time in 1932. The first chairman was Ōshima Tatsujirō,[1] director of Central Hygiene Bureau of the Home Ministry, and the first president was Miyake. From that time on, this council was held every year, and in 1935 was renamed Japan Association of Mental Hospitals.

The Japan Association of Mental Hygiene was originally a private institution, and its official establishment in 1931. Its inaugural ceremony was attended by the then minister of the Home Office. The president was Miyake, and the vice-presidents were Uematsu Shichikurō,[2] Shimoda Mitsuzō, Wada Toyotane,[3] and Marui Kiyoyasu.[4] From 1931, this association published the bulletin *Seishin eisei*[5] [Mental Hygiene], which would have thirty-one issues until 1941. Even after its incorporation into the Association of Mental Welfare, the bulletin continued to exist with the same title, and had one hundred seventeen issues until 1969 when the last one was published. Before the official inauguration of the Association of Mental Hygiene, Miyake had begun to publish the magazine titled *Nō*[6] [Brain], in cooperation with Komine Shigeyuki[7] and Kikuchi Jinichi.[8] This magazine, designed for the public promotion of mental hygiene, continued until 1940, and then with a new title *Seishin to Kagaku*[9] [Mind and Science], until 1944.

After the defeat of the Pacific War, the General Headquarters (GHQ)[10] pointed out the inadequacy of the Mental Patients' Custody Act (1900) and the Mental Hospital Act (1911). On the one hand, the Association of Mental Welfare collaborated with the GHQ for the revision of these laws, and on the other hand, Kaneko Junji drew up a private draft in corporation with Uematsu Shichikurō. As a result, the *Seishineiseihō* [Mental Hygiene Act] was adopted in 1950, abolishing home custody and creating the mental hygiene consultation bureau.[11] Compared with the former Mental Patients' Custody Act, this new law was epoch-making for humanitarian care of the mentally ill. But the character of social protection rested partly, with the stipulation that "protective custody"[12] would be permitted when a patient could not promptly be admitted into a public hospital. It was not until 1965 with the revision of the Mental Hygiene Act that "protective custody" was abolished. In 1964, the U. S. Ambassador Edwin O. Reischauer was stabbed in an assassination attempt, by an adolescent who had undergone outpatient treatment in a mental hospital. This incident caused a great sensation with the phrase "a psychopath at large." In the aftermath, the revision of the act also enforced involuntary confinement in public hospitals. But on the other hand, the revised act introduced a local care system, admitting the public responsibility of payment and the

---

1. 大島辰二郎　　2. 植松七九郎　　3. 和田豊種　　4. 丸井清泰　　5.『精神衛生』
6.『脳』　7. 小峯茂之　　8. 菊地甚一　　9.『精神と科学』
10. 連合国最高司令官総司令部　　11. 精神衛生相談所　　12. 保護拘束

obligation of the public health center concerning mental hygiene. In 1984, some nurses injured a patient resulting in death in Utsunomiya Hospital,[1] and the Japanese psychiatric system came under criticism at the global level due to this incident. In the aftermath of this incident in 1987, the parliament adopted the Mental Health Act, which underlined the defense of human rights and the preparation of a rehabilitation program. This act remains in effect even today.

2. Psychiatrists and Eugenics

As is evident in this outline of psychiatric history, mental hygiene in 20th century Japan had thus developed, with a deep-rooted tendency toward social protection which had already appeared in the Mental Patients' Custody Act of 1900. In such a history, the question remains about how Japanese psychiatry thought about eugenics, including sterilization. First of all, we can easily find some traces of American influence: in 1921, just after the enforcement of the Mental Hospital Act, Martin Barr gave a lecture "Prevention of the Feebleminded"[2] at the Psychiatry Conference in Tokyo, considering the legislation of sterilization which had just started in some states in the U. S. Superintendent of the Elwyn Training School for the Mentally Retarded, he insisted that Japan also needed a sterilization law. Kure attended this conference, but showed a negative attitude toward such a possibility. The Research Committee for Health, mentioned above, soon began to discuss this problem in light of race hygiene. In 1930, a special section on race hygiene was created in this Committee, and in the same year, the Japan Society of Race Hygiene[3] was also established. Its first president was physiologist Nagai Hisomu, and among the secretary members, the name of psychiatrist Miyake Kōichi can be found. As already pointed out, the Research Committee for Health was founded in 1916 with 34 members, including Nagai as well as Miyake. Another member, on whom we will focus later, was Yoshimasu Shūfu,[4] a psychiatrist who especially made a theoretical contribution in the Japan Society of Race Hygiene.

In 1933, just after the establishment of the Nazi regime, Germany enacted the Law for the Prevention of Hereditarily Diseased Offspring.[5] This legislation, which included compulsory sterilization,[6] directly influenced Japan, and caused a strong movement for the enactment of a sterilization law. In 1934, a bill for the Race Eugenic Protection Act was presented to the Imperial Parliament, but failed to be adopted. In 1938, the Ministry of Health and Welfare was founded, and in this ministry, a Eugenic Section was set up under the Prevention Bureau. This section soon started to plan the National Eugenic Act,[7] on the basis of a draft that the Japan Society of Race Hygiene had prepared.

---

1. 宇都宮病院　2.「精神薄弱の予防」　3. 日本民族衛生学会　4. 吉益脩夫
5. 遺伝病子孫予防法　6. 強制断種法　7. 国民優生法

However, this law, adopted in 1940 and enforced in 1941, had no article stipulating compulsory sterilization, which was consequently never practiced. It was after the defeat of the Pacific War, in 1948, that the legislation of compulsory sterilization and compulsory abortion was realized under the Eugenic Protection Law.[1] This was just two years before the legislation of the Mental Hygiene Law, enacted in 1950.

In this period, according to Okada Yasuo, "most of the psychiatrists supported the idea of sterilization, but as it became clear that the draft would permit the use of compulsory sterilization, they began to show a negative attitude toward its legislation." And as psychiatrists who were strongly opposed to sterilization legislation, Okada mentioned the names of Kaneko Junji, Uematsu Shichikurō, Narita Katsurō,[2] and Kikuchi Jin-ichi. Among them, especially Kaneko was strongly opposed, and wrote in just one year of 1938 ten articles opposing sterilization legislation. The reasons for his opposition were as follows: "the real mechanism of heredity about mental disease is not elucidated yet," "sterilization legislation will disturb the progress of medical treatment," "there is not a single cause of mental disease" "there is always uncertainty about diagnosis of disease and evaluation of its severity," "even if sterilization did reduce the frequency of mental diseases, its contribution would be quite limited, and it would be impossible to eradicate mental disease." In an interview which Okada made with Kaneko, the latter stated that sterilization "is like drawing water from the ocean with a cup." Another reason for his opposition to sterilization legislation came from the fact that he had many patients from high society and the imperial family (Okada 2002a, 190-193).

In fact, there was no definitive, uncontested theory concerning the heredity of mental disease then (nor is there today). For various symptoms of disease, there were various points of view and various methods of treatment. For example, Miyake Kōichi, in his article "The characteristics of evil men observed from the psychiatric viewpoint," which was picked up in the bulletin *Eugenics*[3] edited by Gotō Ryūkichi,[4] insisted on inherited criminal tendencies. Although he rejected Lombroso's theory according to which criminals have some recognizable physical features, he accepted the criminals' mental deficiency and their lack of moral and social sense. Such a mental state, said Miyake, largely results from hereditary causes, even if it must be admitted that there is partly some social influence: "Most criminals hereditarily acquire some disposition that causes a reflex response particular to evil men" (Miyake 1928, 14). On the other hand, his article titled "Pathology of Education,"[5] also published in *Eugenics*, came from a lecture on education for "the feebleminded." In this article, Miyake insisted on the necessity of education rather than the influence of heredity. According to him, it is necessary not to correct the demerits of the feebleminded but to promote their merits, for

---

1. 優生保護法　　2. 成田勝郎　　3. 『優生学』　　4. 後藤龍吉　　5. 「教育病理学」

they can be improved by education. And in order to do so, he asserted that a special institution must be established (Miyake 1929). In addition, in "Neurasthenia and mild forms of Psychosis"[1] (originally a lecture given to students at the Tokyo Imperial University in 1936 and partly from his book *Mental Hygiene*),[2] he rejected the theory which considers psychosis, including *dementia praecox*,[3] to be a hereditary disease (Miyake 1936, 131). In another article in the same book, he asserted to the contrary that the feeblemindedness comes from not only "cerebral disease"[4] but also from "heredity." In this way, according to Miyake's viewpoints, what is hereditary is not the disease itself but some tendency toward it, and heredity is not the only cause, but just one among several causes, some of which are acquired.

However, Yoshimasu Shūfu, who took a principal role in psychiatric theorization in the Japan Society of Race Hygiene, insisted more clearly on the heredity of mental disease. He assumed a determined attitude toward the promotion of eugenic practices, including sterilization. Surprisingly, even in the 1960s, he continued to insist firmly on the necessity of eugenics. His *Yūseigaku*[5] [Eugenics], coauthored with other psychiatrists, was published in 1961. Included were photographs of Nagai Hisomu and Miyake Kōichi, who were already deceased at that time and to whom the book was dedicated. It was rewritten from his former *Yuseigaku no riron to jissai*[6] [Theory and Practices of Eugenics] (1940), and he insisted on its continuity with the prewar era, saying that "since the former book was never written to adapt itself to the temporary politics of the government then, there is nothing concerning eugenics theory that requires any modification or revision now" (Yoshimasu 1961, i). And even in 1961, more than fifteen years after the defeat of the war, Yoshimasu showed his firm belief that eugenics was still needed: "in my opinion, the problem of population of the moment has been much discussed in postwar Japan, while the problem of its quality has been much ignored. But considering the peace and welfare of our nation in the future, eugenic problems are too important to be forgotten" (Yoshimasu 1961, i). Yoshimasu thus showed his understanding that the quality[7] rather than quantity[8] of population needed to be addressed in peacetime.

In this way, in his book of 1961, he insisted clearly on the necessity of eugenic sterilization:[9] "in a word, eugenic sterilization is a large-scale plan for the future of our nation, and its importance has not been lost. Today's urgent population policy must be solved on the whole from a eugenic consideration, without which the population policy would leave the root of the problem for thousands of years. Eugenic sterilization is an indispensable tool for the welfare of humankind" (Yoshimasu 1961, 127). And Yoshimasu asserted that even castration[10] could be permitted for some cases, as a "last

1. 「神経衰弱と軽い精神病」 2. 『精神衛生』 3. 早発性痴呆 4. 「脳病」
5. 『優生学』 6. 『優生学の理論と実際』 7. 人口の質 8. 人口の量
9. 優生的断種 10. 去勢

resort" (Yoshimasu 1961, 224). Besides "hard" policies like sterilization and castration, he also recommended "soft" policies like marriage consultation,[1] and underlined the supplementary character of these two kinds of practices: "marriage consultation and sterilization assume a role in practical eugenics like two wheels of a vehicle [which support each other]" (Yoshimasu 1961, 238).

Such strong insistence on eugenics does not seem to be found in Kure Shūzō or Miyake Kōichi. Therefore we cannot consider Yoshimasu Shūfu to be representative of psychiatrists in modern Japan. As already noted, historian Okada points out the fact that some psychiatrists were firmly opposed to the sterilization legislation policy. But Yoshimasu, born in 1899, belonged to a later generation than Kure, born in 1865, and Miyake, born in 1876. The activity span of Yoshimasu's generation crossed over the period of the Pacific war, and it was rather in the postwar era that this generation assumed an influential role in Japanese psychiatry. It can therefore be assumed that there is some specific tendency toward eugenics which is typical of this generation. It will be very important to verify this hypothesis, for such verification will lead to an examination of the continuity between the prewar period and the postwar period and the new development of eugenics related to the period of rapid economic growth in 1950s and 60s. For consideration of such problems, continued research is needed, focusing on other psychiatrists who belonged to the same generation as Yoshimasu.

References

Hashimoto Akira [橋本明]. 2011. *Seishinbyōsha to shitakukanchi* [精神病者と私宅監置 近代日本精神医療史の基礎的研究 Mental Patients and Home Custody]. Tokyo: Rikka Shuppan.

Japanese Society of Mental Health. 2002. *Zusetsu Nihon no seishinhoken undō no ayumi: seishinbyōsha jizenkyūchikai setsuritsu 100 nen kinen* [図説　日本の精神保健運動の歩み―精神病者慈善救治会設立 100 年記念 Illustrated History of Mental Health Movement in Japan]. Tokyo: Nihon Seishin-eiseikai.

Kaneko Junji [金子準二] et al. 1982. *Kaitei/zōho Nihon seishin igaku nenpyō* [改定・増補 日本精神医学年表 A Chronological Table of Psychiatry in Japan]. Tokyo: Makino Shuppan.

Kure Shūzō [呉秀三], Kashida Gorō [樫田五郎]. 2012 (1918). *Seishinbyōsha shitakukanchi no jikkyō* [精神病者私宅監置の実況 Description and Statistical observation of the mentally ill under home custody], contemporary Japanese translation and commentary by Kanekawa Hideo [金川 英雄]. Tokyo: Igaku Shoin.

Miyake Kōichi [三宅鑛一]. 1928. "Seishinbyōgakuteki ni mitaru akunin no tokushitsu" [精神病学的に観たる悪人の特質 The characteristics of evil men observed from the psychiatric

---

1. 結婚相談

viewpoint] in *Yūseigaku* [優生学 Eugenics], edited by Gotō Ryūkichi [後藤龍吉], 5:12, 12-14.
———. 1929. "Kyōikubyōrigaku" [教育病理学 Pathology of Education] in Yūseigaku [優生学 Eugenics], edited by Gotō Ryūkichi 6:6, 27-31.
———. 1933. *Igakuteki shinrigaku* [医学的心理学 Medical Psychology]. Tokyo: Nankodo.
———. 1936. *Seishineisei* [精神衛生 Mental Hygiene]. Tokyo: Teikoku Daigaku Shimbunsha.
Okada Yasuo [園田靖雄]. 2002a. *Nihon seishinka iryōshi* [日本精神科医療史 History of Psychiatric Practice in Japan]. Tokyo: Igaku Shoin.
———. 2002b. "Kokuminyūseihō, Yūseihogohō to seishinka'i" [国民優生法・優生保護法と精神科医 National Eugenic Act, Eugenic Protection Act and Psychiatrists] in *Botai hogohō to watashitachi: chūzetsu, tataigensū, funinshujutsu wo meguru seido to shakai* [母体保護法とわたしたち—中絶・多胎減数・不妊手術をめぐる制度と社会 [Maternal Protection Law and us: abortion, reduction of multiple births, and sterilization—a look at the system and society], edited by Saitō Yukiko [斎藤由紀子]. Tokyo: Akashi Shoten.
Suzuki Akihito [鈴木晃仁]. 2003. "The State, family, and the insane in Japan" in *The Confinement of the Insane: International Perspectives*, 1800-1965, Roy Porter & David Wright, ed. Cambridge: Cambridge University Press.
Suzuki Zenji [鈴木善次]. 1983. *Nihon no yūseigaku: Sono shisō to undō no kiseki* [日本の優生学—その思想と運動の軌跡 Japanese Eugenics: The Legacy of Eugenic Thought and the Eugenics Movement]. Tokyo: Sankyo Shuppan.
Yoshimasu Shūfu [吉益脩夫]. 1940. *Yūseigaku no riron to jissai* [優生学の理論と実際 Theory and Practices of Eugenics]. Tokyo: Nankodo.
———, et al. 1961. *Yūseigaku* [優生学 Eugenics]. Tokyo: Nankodo.

Chapter 3

Eugenic Thought of Abe Isoo, Social Reformer in Japan

Kawashima Sachio

*I*n 1901 the first socialist party in Japan was organized—the Social Democratic Party.[1] Five of its six members were Christians. The founding declaration of the party was drafted by Christian socialist Abe Isoo.[2] The party was prohibited on the day after its founding because it was considered to be of possible danger to the state. Abe remained a parliamentary social democrat with moderate reformism: his final goal was indeed a socialistic society, but he also regarded charitable work and social welfare by the state as instruments to solve the serious social problems caused by capitalism.

The most important social question for Abe was poverty. In face of inadequate charity work and insufficient social policies at that time, he assumed, however, that it was necessary to reduce the large labor population and its reproduction and expected eugenics to achieve this purpose.

1. Outline of Abe Isoo's Life

Abe Isoo was born as the son of a lower samurai on February 4, 1865 in Fukuoka. On recommendation of his brother-in-law, he entered Doshisha English School in Kyoto to learn English. There he was baptized by the founder and president Rev. Niijima Jō[3] and became a Protestant Christian. After his graduation, he worked as the pastor of the Okayama Congregational Church for several years. Between 1891 and 1894, he studied at Hartford Theological Seminary in Connecticut in the United States, observed social work in London, and finally entered the department of theology at Berlin University in Germany. From 1899 Abe taught English and economics at Tokyo College,[4] later Waseda University, founded a student baseball team there, and retired in 1927 at 63 years of age. He continued his study and worked as a statesman of proletarian parties.

Abe researched not only economics and socialism, but was also engaged in political activities. In 1899 he joined the Socialist Society,[5] and became one of the founding members of the Social Democratic Party. After its prohibition, he founded the Social

---

1. 社会民主党　2. 安部磯雄　3. 新島襄　4. 東京専門学校　5. 社会主義協会

Common People's Party[1] which was also prohibited. At the time of the Ashio copper mine poisoning incident,[2] he and his students traveled there and were engaged intensively in relief work for the injured peasants. From 1903 he supported the Commoners' Society[3] of Kōtoku Shūsui,[4] but instead of participating in Kōtoku's direct action, he carried out non-violent legal action.

During the Russo-Japanese War, Abe, influenced by gospel of Jesus and the principle of nonresistance of Russian writer Leo Tolstoy,[5] took an anti-war stance. The principles of pacifism and nonresistance remained his fundamental position until the 1910s. In 1926 he became an advisor for the Labor-Farmer Party,[6] afterwards became the chairman of the Social People's Party,[7] and then president of the Social Mass Party[8] in 1932. At the first general election in 1928, he was elected to the Diet. To show his opposition to Representative Saitō Takao's dismissal from the Diet due to criticism of the military action of the Japanese Army in China, Abe pulled out of his own party in 1940, and then left the Parliament as well when the national mobilization system[9] was introduced at the end of the same year.

But Abe could not continue to hold his anti-war conviction. Already in World War I, he had changed over to support Japanese entry into the war. In the war between China and Japan (1931-1945), he insisted on peace through an alliance of Japan, Manchuria, and China under Japanese leadership, and justified the Japanese aggressive war against Mao Ze-dong's[10] Red Army and Chiang Kai-shek's[11] National Party Army. Abe considered the Pacific War[12] to be defensive action against the American and English "robbers." "For that reason we Japanese must fight to the end until our last man" (Abe 1944, *Kakusei* 34: 5, 2). On September 2, 1945, the war ended with Japan's unconditional surrender. Neither reflection nor repentance about his change from an anti war conviction to the support of Japanese wars can be found in Abe's postwar remarks.

Immediately after the War, a proposal to found a united socialist party was announced by Abe Isoo, Kagawa Toyohiko,[13] and Takano Iwasaburō,[14] with the formation of the Japan Socialist Party[15] in November 1945. In the general election in 1947, this party won the largest number of seats. Christian socialist lawyer Katayama Tetsu,[16] one of Abe's juniors, became Prime Minister. On February 10, 1949, Abe died in Tokyo at the age of 84, and his funeral service was performed at the Fujimichō Church.*1

1. 社会平民党   2. 足尾銅山鉱毒事件   3. 平民社   4. 幸徳秋水
5. レオ・トルストイ   6. 労働農民党   7. 社会民衆党   8. 社会大衆党
9. 国家総動員体制   10. 毛沢東   11. 蔣介石   12. 太平洋戦争   13. 賀川豊彦
14. 高野岩三郎   15. 日本社会党   16. 片山哲

2. Abe Isoo's Christianity

Rev. Niijima Jō, who baptized Abe Isoo, returned to Japan in 1874 as a Congregational missionary after his study in the United States. Niijima's faith was orthodox: creation of everything by God, human sin, redemption by the cross of Jesus Christ, the Son of God and his resurrection, repentance of the sinner, the Trinity (Father, Son, and Holy Spirit), etc. After Abe graduated from Doshisha and was not under Niijima's direct influence, his belief shifted to Unitarianism. Also called "New Theology," it denies both the godhood of Jesus and the doctrine of the Trinity and respects Jesus only as the highest moral teacher. One should obey him and live a pure, moral life. One does not need to believe in the miracles and "unscientific" stories of the Bible, but should interpret the contents and understand the meanings behind the stories. Abe's new convictions were established during his study in Berlin, Germany.

Abe belonged to the Unitarian Society[1] in Japan. Its members attached importance to a moral way of life rather than repentance of sin. Abe often wrote essays for *Rikugō Zasshi*[2] [Universe Magazine], the publication of Japanese Unitarians. His maxim— "Simple Life and High Ideals"—shows a Unitarian character. The Unitarian Society of Japan, however, stood in opposition to American Unitarians, and dispersed after the Tokyo Earthquake of 1923 (See Abe 1932 and Wakagi 1966).

3. Abe Isoo's Socialism

During his stay at Hartford Theological Seminary, Abe Isoo read Edward Bellamy's[3] 1888 utopian novel *Looking Backward 2000-1887* and became a socialist. After he had observed various kinds of social work in America and England, he concluded that it was not easy to solve social problems by social work. Bellamy's novel impressed him deeply, and he came to believe in a socialistic future.

According to Abe, the most serious problem produced by capitalism was poverty caused by the unequal distribution of wealth. He listed five ways to try to solve the poverty question:
1) Relief work: charities and social work
2) Educational work: social education and settlements
3) Social policy: social insurance, legislation for protection of workers, tax reform
4) Civil organizations: trade unions, associations, guilds and co-operatives
5) Socialism: socialization and equal distribution of the means of production, banks, transport, electricity

1. ユニテリアン協会   2. 『六合雑誌』   3. エドワード・ベラミー

Abe regarded the ways 1) through 4) as significant, but saw socialism as the fundamental solution to reach the final goal. However, his method for reaching this goal was not by direct actions like general strikes and violent revolution, but by moderate reform through parliamentary actions. Abe rejected Marxism and syndicalism and supported a social democracy as in England. The Social Democratic Party of Germany,[1] which had gained a large number of seats in the Parliament at that time, was the model of a socialist party for him (See Abe 1932; Matsuo 2010; Nakamura 1969; Okamoto 2001; Tsujino 1983; Yamaizumi 1981).

4. Eugenic Thought of Abe Isoo

a) Poverty[2] as the center of social problems

In his representative book *Shakai mondai gairon*[3] [Outline of Social Problems, 1921], Abe paid great attention to the population problem in order to solve contemporary social questions. He acknowledged that a direct method to help the poor could be indeed helpful to provide relief for the poor, but that there was not being enough accomplished at that time. The impoverished would need to reduce their population themselves. A large population of workers, for example, decreases workers' wages, causes unemployment, and results in poverty in the end. Poverty was the main cause of another population problem—the destitution of farmers, who made up over half of the total population of Japan at the time. He concluded that, in general, the more the number of children increases, the poorer each home becomes economically, regardless of profession (Abe 1921, 665-672).

According to Abe, a nation with a superfluous population tends to try to expand its territory and wage war in order to export its own people. One assumes that the development of a nation needs to increase the population, but that is false. The number of children must be decreased through birth control, and an effort must be made to strengthen the quality rather than the quantity of the nation. "Our nation must make more effort for human betterment than for armament." It is necessary to try reducing births and rearing of our children wisely. "Human betterment is the most effective way to conquer poverty" (Abe 1921, 677).

b) Birth control, eugenics and sterilization

Concerning birth control, Abe had high praise for eugenics, which was spreading among Japanese intellectuals. "It is eugenically the most proper method to have superior men continue to bear offspring and to have men with bad heredity limit their offspring. ... It is only natural to control persons of inferior quality to some degree for the happiness of

1. ドイツ社会民主党   2. 貧困   3. 『社会問題概論』

all mankind" (Abe 1921, 673).

How was eugenic birth control put into practice in Japan? Abe, leader of the birth control movement[1] in Japan from the 1920s, regarded not only voluntary birth control by citizens as necessary, but also regarded state legislation of sterilization[2] and execution of eugenic policy as important. "It is necessary for the state to attempt some intervention in the [private lives of its] citizens in order to achieve the purpose of race betterment. In other words, intervention which makes superior heredity possible by the power of legislation should never be opposed" (Abe 1921, 683).

Abe insisted that the marriage of persons with bad heredity should be restricted and wrote that several states in America "prohibit the marriages of the desperately poor, ... idiots, epileptics, and the mentally ill, and there are other places that prohibit the marriages of alcoholics and habitual criminals." Because of this, he felt there was merit in having a couple exchange documents issued by a physician certifying their health before marriage (Abe 1921, 684ff). Referring to instances of some states in America, he regarded sterilization laws as especially important.

> Since 1907 the number of states in America which have passed legislation to prevent reproduction has reached twelve.... These laws apply to persons interned in state prisons, mental hospitals, or institutions for idiots.... In Indiana, a committee composed of three surgeons determines whether or not the law should be carried out on persons with bad heredity (Abe 1921, 686ff).

Abe also wrote that the state should segregate such weak persons in order to protect them from society's competition (Abe 1921, 687f).

In his book *Sanji seigen ron*[3] [Theory of Birth Restriction, 1922], Abe wrote that the reasons for his opinion were the bad effects of multiple births on mothers' health, prevention of the deformed and disabled, and the prevention of an increase in hereditary diseases. "It is our obligation to send out into society children who are better than we. On the contrary, I think it is the worst crime for us to send out inferior descendants into society." But he did not yet mention sterilization in this book. Abe insisted that birth restriction was necessary to realize world peace and the emancipation of women (Abe 1922, 155, 167).

In another representative book, *Seikatsu mondai kara mita sanji chōsetsu*[4] [Birth control seen from lifestyle problems, 1931], Abe explained concrete birth control methods, especially sterilization. He recommended male sterilization, that is, vasectomy in following cases: if a family has already seven or eight children and wants no more, if

---

1. 産児調節運動　2. 断種（不妊手術，優生手術）　3. 『産児制限論』
4. 『生活問題から見た産児調節』

the wife is in poor health, if the family has two or three deformed children, if the parent is afflicted with mental disease, disability, or hereditary disease. Vasectomy[1] is an easy surgical operation. Abe wrote, "I recommend this method from viewpoint of eugenics," and leprosy[2] patients should be permitted to be married on the condition of undergoing this operation (Abe 1931, 233f).

To justify his opinion, Abe referred to the "Report to Home Minister about Race Hygiene" of the Japan Medical Association[3] in 1928 and presented its plan of legislation affirmatively. According to the report, patients of bad heredity, the disabled, sexual perverts, and habitual criminals could undergo birth control or sterilization. In the case of a ruling by a screening committee, they would have to accept these measures (Abe 1931, 234ff). In the monthly of the League for Birth Control Movement,[4] Abe wrote that such a situation was desirable and that it could be expected that sterilization legislation would be made in the near future and accomplish "the real happiness and interests of the masses" (Abe 1929, 3; see also Fujino 2000; Hatakenaka 2000, 2001; Hayashi 2005, 2009; Mamiya 1993; Sugiyama 1998, 2003).

c) Motivation for acceptance of eugenics

Since when did Abe advocate eugenic thought? Abe wrote in his book for a cultivated life *Risō no Hito*[5] [Ideal Person 1906], "it is most important to nurture a strong and healthy body in one's youth" (Abe 1906, Chap.3: *Kyoiku*[6] [Education], 77). In addition, he also emphasized consideration and education for crippled persons. But at the same time, he asserted: "It is proper to prohibit heavy drinkers and persons of hereditary or epidemic diseases from marriage... by law as in some countries…. They should live as singles if they respect themselves and their descendants" (Abe 1906, Chap. 4,: *Katei*[7] [Home], 28). In his book *Fujin no Risō*[8] [Ideals of Women 1910], he emphasized the ideal women's role in the home and in society and the parity of men and women. He wrote: "It is very wrong to despise dull-witted persons; ...one must have great sympathy for them." "Society has an obligation to provide special educational facilities for disabled children" (Abe 1910, 80). But on the other hand, he wrote: "Is it not Heaven's vengeance for a mother's sin to give birth to an idiot or a mad child, while a perfect offspring is the pride of a mother?" (Abe 1910, 69). Therefore "physical examinations before marriage are necessary... one should get a physician's medical certificate" (Abe 1910, 83).

Abe began then to use the word "eugenics" from the 1910s. In his article "*Nora to Maguda*" (Nora and Magda, 1912) he wrote, "In recent science, the most significant subject of study is eugenics, that is, the race problem. It is of vital importance for us to think about how we can improve our whole race" (Abe 1912, *Kakusei*[9] 2:7, 6).

1. 精管切除（ヴァゼットミー）   2. ハンセン病   3. 日本医師会
4. 産児制限運動連盟   5. 『理想の人』   6. 「教育」   7. 「家庭」   8. 『婦人の理想』
9. 『廓清』

d) Influence of American eugenics

It seems that one motivation for Abe's acceptance of eugenics was eugenic information from America related to the birth control movement to which he strongly committed himself (Hayashi 2009, 37). He wrote an English essay for the American birth control magazine about the Japanese birth control movement in 1923 (Abe 1923).

It was necessary for him, however, to get information and knowledge from his American friends in order to publicize his opinion about eugenics with confidence, especially concerning sterilization. It is here that a direct influence of American eugenics can be seen. The wife of American missionary Horace E. Coleman[1] had introduced Abe to her friend Ezra S. Gosney[2] in the 1920s. Gosney sent many papers about American eugenics and sterilization to Abe, who visited him and Paul Popenoe[3] in the suburbs of Los Angeles in 1929. During that visit, he collected a great deal of eugenic information. Lawyer Gosney impressed Abe as an "enviably splendid person." Gosney entrusted biologist Popenoe with eugenic research. Abe wrote:

> Twenty years have already passed since the legislation of voluntary sterilization in California. About 6000 persons were sterilized—half of them were men. ... The results of the operations were good generally. ... Sterilization in some American states is compulsory for certain persons, for instance, alcoholics and habitual criminals. It is natural, I think, to sterilize persons of bad heredity... because there is no other method for human betterment.

Abe's opinion reached a peak: "Opponents of sterilization of eugenics are enemies of humanity" [!] (Abe 1931b).

After this impressive visit to Gosney and Popenoe, Abe translated their book *Sterilization for Human Betterment* into Japanese. The title avoided the word "sterilization" and used "*Funin-kekkon*,"[4] which in Japanese means "barren marriage or marriage without children in future" (Abe 1930).

e) Presentation of Nazi Germany's Sterilization Law

In 1933 Adolf Hitler[5] became Prime Minister in Germany, and the National Socialist Government enacted a compulsory sterilization law in July—the Law for the Prevention of Hereditarily Diseased Offspring.[6] Its outline was introduced immediately in the magazine *Sanji chōsetsu*,[7] the publication of the Japan Birth Control League for which Abe served as honorary president. The anonymous article was entitled "Extermination of the socially unfit—Execution by national power—Nazi stories"[8] and read as follows:

---

1. ホレイス・E. コールマン　2. エズラ・S. ガスニー　3. ポール・ポペノー
4. 『不妊結婚と人間改造』　5. アドルフ・ヒトラー
6. 遺伝病子孫予防法（ナチス断種法）　7. 『産児調節』
8. 社会不適者を絶滅―国家権力を以って強行―但しナチスの話

The social policies of Hitler in Germany are observed with surprise from all quarters. One of them is about the execution of a new interesting law from January 1 next year, which intends to exterminate offspring who are unfit for life in society. That means a realization of eugenic ideal.

The aim of this law is to compulsorily prevent the probable reproduction of those with the following conditions which are hereditarily unfit from the medical viewpoint of today: inherited epilepsy, schizophrenia, hereditary Huntington's chorea, congenital feeble-mindedness, manic-depressive insanity, hereditary blindness and deafness, hereditary deformity, incurable alcoholism,[1] etc.

Its prevention of probable reproduction (sterilization) is an easy operation which does not diminish sexual feeling. Its method is binding semen or fallopian tubes. This operation may be applied for by patients themselves, by a physician in the district, or by a clinic director.

The application is received by a Eugenic Health Court[2] (*Erbgesundheitsgericht*) consisting of a judge, a medical officer, and a doctor familiar with genetics. This court decides whether the operation is ordered or refused.

However, this law eliminates unhealthy elements from the nation. From a national standpoint it is nothing more than a passive measure." (Abe 1933 *Sanji chōsetsu* 6:8, 63).

Three years later, Abe commented on this law positively, because he had already affirmed compulsory sterilization from a eugenic viewpoint.

In Germany Hitler is recommending sterilization for race betterment. Persons with bad hereditary diseases, persons of low intelligence, persons who will pass on bad genes to their offspring, etc... shall be compulsorily sterilized by state law.... There is no other method so practical (Abe 1936).

f) Eugenic legislation and Hansen's disease

The information about American and European sterilization laws, especially those of Nazi Germany, greatly influenced the promoters and supporters of eugenic legislation in Japan. In the 1930s several draft laws which had regulations about the sterilization of persons with mental or hereditary disease had been proposed in the Parliament without success. In this situation on December 17, 1939, Abe Isoo was invited as speaker to a meeting on race hygiene research which was organized by the Race Hygiene Group in the Eugenic Division of the Disease Prevention Department in the Ministry of Health and

---

1. 遺伝性のてんかん，精神分裂病，遺伝性ハンチントン病，先天性の精神薄弱，そううつ病，遺伝性の盲，聾，遺伝性の不具，不治のアルコール中毒
2. 優生裁判所（遺伝健康裁判所）

Welfare[1]. Based on memories of his visit to American eugenicists Gosney and Popenoe, he stated that sterilization laws had been enacted and were already being carried out in 29 of the 48 American states. "It is good that this problem is now being actively discussed, and this legislation will soon be in our country too." He left the matter of drafting a sterilization law to other experts and turned his attention to the problem of Hansen's disease.

> I think that the most urgent problem which we must tackle... is the case of leprosy. ... Isn't it quite merciless that leprosy patients are forbidden to be married? It is grievous, of course, if they were to give birth. I think it is only natural to permit them to marry on the condition that they are sterilized to bear no children."

Abe praised Dr. Mitsuda Kensuke,[2] Director of the Nagashima Sanatorium[3] who was sterilizing leprous patients even though it was illegal.*[2]

g) National Eugenic Law and Kagawa Toyohiko

In 1940 the National Eugenic Law,[4] which Abe had long awaited, was passed. This law regulated the sterilization of persons with diseases similar to those in the Nazi German Sterilization Law. However, the Japanese law made only voluntary sterilization possible and excluded the sterilization of alcoholics and habitual criminals (see Kawashima 2006 and 2013). The execution of compulsory sterilization (Article 6) was suspended, because Japan needed an increase in population for the impending war. The slogan at that time was "Be fruitful and multiply!"[5]

I could not find any comments by Abe about the National Eugenic Law. But there is no doubt from his opinion, as in the past, that he welcomed this sterilization law. For a hint concerning his opinion, I refer to a comment of pastor Kagawa Toyohiko, who was also an active social reformer and representative leader of Protestantism in Japan. He wrote an article: "*Yūseihō to bosei no shūkyōteki jikaku*"[6] [Eugenic law and religious responsibility for maternity] in his magazine *Kumo no Hashira*[7] [Pillar of Cloud] soon after the enactment of the new law:

> Recently in Japan a new good law was passed. The Eugenic Law was enacted in Parliament and is about to be carried out. This Law intends mainly to exterminate bad heredity which is harmful to the state and to save our life from such heredity. That is indeed a desirable law (Kagawa 1940, 12).

Kagawa assumed, like Abe, that " idiocy, disability, madness, and perversion are

---

1. 厚生省予防局優生課　2. 光田健輔　3. 長島愛生園　4. 国民優生法
5. 「産めよ殖やせよ」　6. 優生法と母性の宗教的自覚　7. 『雲の柱』

hereditary in character" (Kagawa 1947, 5).*³

h) Abe's conversion to the opinion for increase in population

Although Abe continued to support the restriction of population and birth control in the 1920s and sterilization as its means in the 1930s, he did an about-face during the Pacific War¹ (1941-1945), because a different propaganda storm was blowing in all of Japan—"Be fruitful and multiply!" He suddenly began to assert a new appeal for an increase in population:

> Japan is facing a critical moment now.... For waging war, the more population we have, the more advantageous it is.... Although our opinion about the population problem was negative previously, we now think that a larger population is necessary for victory in the World War. But only increasing the number of people is not enough, we must better the quality of individuals. Only increasing the numbers is useless if the quality is not good" (Abe 1943).

So we can say that Abe's eugenic thought never vanished even throughout the war.

As Japan's defeat neared, Abe believed the reports of Japanese newspapers that America's war aim was the extermination of the Japanese.

> In order to achieve that goal, it is best to use the strength of the law to physiologically castrate all Japanese males. That would make it possible to bring an end to the Japanese race. If that is not done, the British and the Americans can never spend their days in peace." (Abe 1944).

i) Return to population restriction, birth control, and the Eugenic Protection Law

In 1945 Japan lost the war, and many soldiers returned to their homeland. The birth rate increased rapidly despite the lack of food. The voice of caution against surplus population¹ became loud, and the appeal for restriction of population and birth control was revived. Abe Isoo, now over 80 years old, returned to his former position, that is, as an opinion leader of less population and birth control.

> If a race has surplus population, it will inevitably be an element which disrupts peace.... It is a natural obligation for a peaceful race to keep a reasonable scale of population. People defeated in war need to control their population themselves in order to find a way of self-support" (Abe 1948).

1. 過剰人口

In 1948 when he wrote this article, the Eugenic Protection Law[1] was enacted in Parliament. It was the law which made voluntary and compulsory sterilization possible not only for the mentally disabled, insane patients, and persons of hereditary diseases, but also for Hansen's disease patients. This law made it possible to carry out a far stronger eugenic policy than the former National Eugenic Law (See Kawashima 2006).

I did not find any materials which recorded Abe's comments about this Eugenic Protection Law which was passed in the year prior to his death. But we can easily guess that this new law would have been welcomed by him, because he had not given up his eugenic thought even after the War. By way of suggestion, I refer again to a comment of Kagawa, famous Christian Socialist, in the year after the enactment of this law:

> It is a necessary obligation not only for parents but also for society... to restrict the birth of bad hereditary offspring. It is better for the disabled not to be born than to live a miserable life.... It is the wisest method which has been practiced since olden times in Europe to cut the male semen pipes in order to make birth of offspring impossible. I know a kind doctor, Mr. Mitsuda Kensuke, in Japan who also performs operations of cutting semen pipes for leprosy patients in order to prevent infection in the uterus" (Kagawa 1949).

Conclusion

Abe Isoo remained a Christian until his death. He was an honest Christian who consistently practiced a puritan way of life. From his youth, he criticized the vices and contradictions of capitalism and sought a way for socialism's conquest over capitalism through moderate parliamentarianism. Civil and social human rights were oppressed in Japan during his lifetime. Both Christianity and socialism were suspected and regarded as heretical, or even traitorous. It would not have been so easy to dare to live as a Christian Socialist as we might suppose. We need to consider the restrictions of the era, therefore, when we analyze Abe's thought and activities.

Why did he continue to advocate eugenic thought in his whole life? One reason for this may be found in his way of Christian faith. The characteristic substance of Christian doctrine is as follows: God's creation of the world, belief in God only and refusal to make idols of creatures, human's fundamental sin, consciousness of one's own sin and repentance for it, redemption of human sin and salvation by Christ, and then human faith and activity as response to God's grace and love. But Jesus was for Abe the highest and greatest moral model, but not God Himself. It was important for him that we human

---

1. 優生保護法

beings live purely and rightly, and a person with a healthy and strong body and soul was his "ideal person." Persons with incurable or hereditary diseases, mental defects, etc. should not have been born. For him, the way to realize this aim was through birth control and/or sterilization.

According to his conviction, unhealthy children cause unhappiness for themselves, for their families, and for society, and they have a fundamental right not to be born. Only an immoral person would bear such children.[*4]

Such eugenic thought is never just a story of the past. What aim do the recent prenatal tests[1] on a mother's body have? They offer a choice to the parents whether to give birth or not, after inspecting hereditary genes of the coming baby. Then we can say that we also live today with our own eugenic thought, although it may come neither from misunderstanding of Christian faith like Abe's, nor from state law.

Finally, I would like to say just a word about my estimation of Abe Isoo. My analysis of his problematic points does not mean totally denying his many good intentions and results of his ideas and actions. I would like to confirm only that he was an ordinary person, just like those whom he esteemed lowly, with his own share of sins, faults, and fundamental weaknesses. He failed to understand Jesus' teaching about the importance of "the least of these" (Matthew 25:40).

Notes

*1 See Abe 1932; *Abe Isoo no Kenkyū* 1990; Iguchi 2011; Katayama 1958; Miyamoto 1984; Powles 1978; Takano 1970. About Abe's conversion from pacifism to pro-war sympathy see Izuhara 2000 and 2007; Nakamura Naomi 1987 and 1989; Okamoto 2002; Ōta 1975.

*2 *Minzoku Eisei Shiryō* ［民族衛生資料 Materials of Race Hygiene］ 6 (Mar. 1939), 1-6 in *Sei to Seishoku no Jinkenmondai Shiryō Shūsei*, 26, 316-319. See also Fujino 2000 and Sugiyama 1998 and 2003.

*3 About Kagawa Toyohiko see Kawashima 1985, 1988 and 1991; Schildgen 1988. About his eugenic thought see Fujino 2000, Sugiyama 1998, 2003 and 2010.

*4 For a significant analysis of Abe Isoo's Christian faith, see Wakagi 1966, and for an interesting paper about Abe's eugenic thought, see Hayashi 2005 and 2009.

References

Abe Isoo ［安部磯雄］. 1900. "Shakaishugisha to shite no Kirisuto" ［社会主義者としての基督 Christ as Socialist］ in *Rikugō Zasshi* ［六合雑誌］ 232, 52-57.

―――. 1901. *Shakaimondai Kaishakuhō* ［社会問題解釈法 How to solve social problems］. Tokyo: Waseda Daigaku Shuppanbu.

1. 出生前診断

——. 1906. *Risō no Hito* ［理想の人 Ideal person］. Tokyo: Ryokodo.
——. 1910. *Fujin no Risō* ［婦人の理想 Ideals of Women］. Tokyo: Hokubunkan.
——. 1921. *Shakaimondai Gairon* ［社会問題概論 Outline of social problems］. Tokyo: Waseda Daigaku Shuppanbu.
——. 1922. *Sanji seigen ron* ［産児制限論 Theory of Birth Restriction］. Tokyo: Jitsugyo no Nipponsha.
——. 1923. "The Birth Control Movement in Japan" in *The Birth Control Review* 7:1, 9, 17.
——. 1927. *Jinkō mondai to sanji seigen* ［人口問題と産児制限 Population problem and Birth Restriction］. Tokyo: Keimeisha.
—— and Majima Kan ［馬島僩］. 1925. *Sanji seigen no riron to jissai* ［産児制限の理論と実際 Theory and practice of birth restriction］. Tokyo: Bunkagakkai Shuppanbu.
——. 1929. "Tada taishū no kōfuku aru nomi" ［唯大衆の幸福あるのみ Only the happiness of the masses is important］ in *Sanji seigen* ［産児制限 Birth Control］ 2:1 (Jan.), 3 reprinted in *Sei to seishoku no jinkenmondai shiryō shūsei* 2001, 13, 63.
——. (Translation) 1930. *Funin kekkon to ningen kaizō* ［不妊結婚と人間改造 Sterilization for Human Betterment］ by E. S. Gosney and Paul Popenoe. New York: Macmillan 1929). Tokyo: Shunyodo.
——. 1931. *Seikatsu mondai kara mita sanji chōsetu* ［生活問題から見た産児調節 Birth control seen from lifestyle problems］. Tokyo: Tokyodo.
——. 1931b. "Sanjiseigen no yūseigakuteki kenkai" ［産児制限の優生学的見解 Eugenic Opinion on birth restrictionl］ in *Sanji chōsetu* ［産児調節 Birth Control］ 4:5 (June) 2-5. Reprinted in *Sei to seishoku no jinkenmondai shiryō shūsei* 13, 335f.
——. 1932. *Shakaishugisha to naru made* ［社会主義者となるまで Until I became a socialist］. Tokyo: Kaizosha.
——. 1936. "Kokumin seikatsu to jinkō mondai" ［国民生活と人口問題 National life and the population problem］ in *Kakusei* 26:5 (May), 3.
——. 1943. "Senjika no kekkon mondai" ［戦時下の結婚問題 Marriage Problem in wartime］ in *Kakusei* 33:4 (April), 2
——. 1944. "Kokumin no kakugo" ［国民の覚悟 The preparedness of citizens］ in *Kakusei: The Purity* 34: 5, 2.
——. 1948. "Sanjichōsetsu undō no hatten no tame ni" ［産児調節運動の発展のために For the development of birth control movement］ in *Sanchō jihō* ［産調時報 The Birth Control News］ 1 (Nov.), 2. Reprinted in *Sei to seishoku no jinkenmondai shiryō shūsei* 14, 5, 7.
——. 2008. *Abe Isoo chosakushū* ［安部磯雄著作集　全6巻　Abe Isoo Selected Works Vol.1-6］. Tokyo: Ronsosha.
Abe Isoo Kenkyū bukai ［安部磯雄研究部会］. 1990. *Abe Isoo no Kenkyū*. ［安部磯雄の研究 Study of Abe Isoo］. Tokyo: Waseda Daigaku Shakaikagaku Kenkyusho.

Abe Isoo Nikki Honkoku Iinkai, ed.［安部磯雄日記翻刻委員会］. 2009. *Abe Isoo Nikki: Seishun Hen*［安部磯雄日記—青春編 Abe Isoo's Diary: Youth］in *Extra of Neesima Studies* No.100.

Bellamy, Edward. 1887. *Looking Backward 2000-1887*. New York: Random House. (Japanese Translation by Yamamoto Masaki［山本政喜］1953/1986 *Kaeri mireba*［顧りみれば］. Tokyo: Iwanami Bunko.)

Doshisha Sanmyaku Henshū Iinkai, ed.［［同志社山脈編集委員会］. 2003. *Doshisha Sanmyaku*［同志社山脈 The Prominent of Doshisha］, 170f. Kyoto: Koyo Shobo.

Fujino Yutaka［藤野豊］. 2000. *Nihon Fashizumu to Yuseishisō*［日本ファシズムと優生思想 Japanise Fascism and Eugenic Thought］. Kyoto: Kamogawa Shuppan.

Hatakenaka Akiko［畠中暁子］. 2000. "*Kakusei* ni okeru yūseishisō no eikyō to rongi no tenkai［『廓清』における優生思想の影響と論議の展開 Development of the opinion about the influence of Eugenics in *Kakusei*］ in *Kirisutokyō shakaimondai kenkyū*［キリスト教社会問題研究 Study of Christianity and Social problems］49, 122-143.

———. 2001. "*Kakusei* ni okeru sanji chōsetsuron no tenkai"［『廓清』における産児調節論の展開 The development of the birth control argument in *Kakusei*］in *Kirisutokyō shakaimondai kenkyū* 50, 73-94.

Hayashi Yōko［林葉子］. 2005. "Haishōron to sanjiseigenron no yūgō"［廃娼論と産児制限論の融合—安部磯雄の優生思想について The Connection between "Haishō" Theory and Birth Control Theory: the eugenics of Abe Isoo］in *Josei Gaku*（女性学 Journal of Women's Studies）13, 94-110.

———. 2009. "Abe Isoo ni okeru 'heiwa' ron to danshu ron: Danseisei no mondai to no kakawari wo jiku ni"［安部磯雄における「平和」論と断種論 On the Notion of 'Peace' and Sterilization in Abe Isoo: Concerning the Problem of Manliness］in *Jendā Shigaku*［ジェンダー史学］5:35-49.

Hosoi Isamu［細井勇］. 2010. "Abe Isoo: '*Shakaimondai kaishakuhō*' to shakaimondai ron"［安部磯雄—『社会問題解釈法』と社会問題論 Abe Isoo: How to resolve the social problems and Theory of Social Problems］in *Jinbutsu de yomu shakaifukushi no shisō to riron*［人物で読む社会福祉の思想と理論 Reading about ideas and theories from men of social welfare］, Murota Yasuo, ed., 47-53. Kyoto: Minerva Shobo.

Iguchi Takashi［井口隆史］. 2011. *Abe Isoo no shōgai: shisso no seikatsu, kōen no risō*［安部磯雄の生涯—質素之生活　高遠之理想 Life of Abe Isoo: Simple Life, High Ideal］. Tokyo: Waseda Daigaku Shuppanbu.

Izuhara Masao［出原政雄］. 2000. "Daiichiji taisenki ni okeru Abe Isoo no heiwashisō"［第一次大戦期における安部磯雄の平和思想 Abe Isoo's pacifism in WWI］in *Shigakukan hōgaku*［志学館法学 Shigakukan Law Review］1:1, 109-128.

———. 2007. "Heiwashisō no anten"［平和思想の暗転—十五年戦争期の安部磯雄 The enigmatic conversion of Abe Isoo's pacifism in wartime］in *Doshisha hogaku*［同志社法学 The

Doshisha Law Review〕 59:2, 281-311.

Kagawa Toyohiko［賀川豊彦］. 1940. "Yūseihō to bosei no shūkyōteki jikaku"［優生法と母性の宗教的自覚 Eugenic Law and Religious Responsibility for maternity］ in *Kumo no Hashira*［雲の柱 Pillar of Cloud］ 19 (Oct.), 12-15 and 19.

―――. 1947. "Nihon ni okeru shakaijigyō no genzai oyobi shōrai"［日本に於ける社会事業の現在及将来 Social Work Today and Future in Japan］ in *Sekai kokka*［世界国家 World Nation］ 1:3-4, 3-10.

―――. 1949. "Sanji chōsetsu ron"［産児調節論 On Birth Control］ in *Sekai kokka* 3:4 (May), 15-17.

Kakuseikai 1995. *Kakusei*［廓清 The Purity］. Reprint. Tokyo: Fuji Shuppan.

Katayama Tetsu［片山哲］. 1958. *Abe Isoo Den*［安部磯雄伝 A Biography of Abe Isoo］ Tokyo: Mainichi Shimbunsha.

Kawashima Sachio［河島幸夫］. 1985. "Toyohiko Kagawa: Christlicher Sozialreformer und Friedenspraktiker" in *Zeichen der Zeit* 39 (April), 98-101.

―――. 1988. *Kagawa Toyohiko no shōgai to shisō*［賀川豊彦の生涯と思想 Life and Thought of Kagawa Toyohiko］. Fukuoka: Nakagawa Shoten.

―――. 1991. *Kagawa Toyohiko to taiheiyō sensō: sensō, heiwa, zaiseki kokuhaku*［賀川豊彦と太平洋戦争―戦争・平和・罪責告白 Toyohiko Kagawa and the Pacific War: War, Peace and Confession of sin］. Fukuoka: Nakagawa Shoten.

―――. 2006. "Botai hogohō no Nachisuteki keifu?"［母体保護法のナチス的系譜？ A genealogy of the Maternal Protection Law?］ in *The Seinan Law Review*［西南学院大学法学論集］ 48:3-4 (Feb.), 1-33.

―――. 2013. "Nachisu yūsei seisaku to Nihon he no eikyō: Idenbyō shison yobohō kara Kokumin Yūseihō e"［ナチス優生政策と日本への影響―遺伝病子孫予防法から国民優生法へ Influence of Nazi Eugenic Policy on Japan: From the Law for Prevention of Hereditarily Deseased Offspring to the National Eugenic Law］ in *Seimei no Rinri 3: Yūsei Seisaku no keifu*［生命の倫理 3 優生政策の系譜 Ethics of Life 3］, Yamazaki Kiyoko, ed., 193-222. Fukuoka: Kyushu Daigaku Shuppankai.

Kubota Eisuke［久保田英助］. 2008. "Abe Isoo no Kakuseikai ni yoru haishō undō no tokushitsu"［安部磯雄の廓清会による廃娼運動の特質―1920 年代における買売春をめぐる日本人の「男性性」Characteristics of Antiprostitution Movement by Abe Isoo's *Kakuseikai*］ in *Ajia bunka kenkyū*［アジア文化研究 Journal of Asian Culture Society］ 15:15, 27-39.

Mamiya Kunio［間宮國夫］. 1993. "Abe Isoo to iminjinkō mondai"［安部磯雄と移民人口問題 Abe Isoo and the Immigration Problem］ in *Shakai kagaku tōkyū*［社会科学討究 The Social Science Review］ 39:1, 27-46.

Matsuo Takayoshi［松尾尊兊］. 2010. *Waga kindai Nihon jinbutsushi*［わが近代日本人物誌 My Study of Modern Japanese Persons］. Tokyo: Iwanami Shoten, 2-14.

Miyamoto Seitarō［宮本盛太郎］. 1984. *Shūkyōteki Ningen no Seijishisō: Abe Isoo to Kanokogi Kazunobu no baai*［宗教的人間の政治思想：安部磯雄と鹿子木員信の場合 Political Ideas of Religious Persons: The case of Abe Isoo and Kanokogi Kazunobu］. Tokyo: Bokutakusha.

Nakamura Katsunori［中村勝範］. 1969. *Meiji shakaishugi kenkyū*［明治社会主義研究 A Study of Meiji Socialism］. Tokyo: Sekai Shoin, 82-116.

Nakamura Naomi［中村尚美］. 1987. "Abe Isoo no hisenron"［安部磯雄の非戦論 Pacifism of Abe Isoo］ in *Shakai kagaku tōkyū*［社会科学討究 The Social Science Review］ 33:2, 1-30.

――――. 1989. "Abe Isoo to jūgonen sensō"［安部磯雄と十五年戦争 Abe Isoo and World War II］ in *Shakai kagaku tōkyū* 34:3, 177-210.

Nihon Kirisutokyō Rekishi Daijiten［日本キリスト教歴史大辞典 History of Christianity in Japan: A Great Encyclopedia］. 1988. Tokyo: Kyobunkan.

Okamoto Hiroshi［岡本宏］. 1970. "Manshū jihen to musan seitō"［満州事変と無産政党 Manchurian Incident and Proletarian Parties］ in *Kokusai seiji*［国際政治 International Politics］ 43, 100-118.

――――. 2002. Abe Isoo: Heiwaron to kokkaron no zeijakusei［安部磯雄―平和論と国家論の脆弱性 Abe Isoo: Fragility of His Peace and State Theory］ in *Kurume Daigaku Hōgaku*［久留米大学法学 The Kurume Law Review］ 45, 25-52.

Ōta Masao［太田雅夫］ 1975. *Taishō demokurashi kenkyū: Chishikijin no shisō to undō*［大正デモクラシー研究―知識人の思想と運動 A Study of Taisho Democracy: Ideas and Movement of the Intellectuals］ 290-319. Tokyo: Shinsensha.

Powles, Cyril H. 1978. "Abe Isoo: The Utility Man" in *Pacifism in Japan: The Christian and Socialist Tradition,* Nobuya Bamba and John F. Howes, ed., 143-167 and 281-287. Kyoto: Minerva Shobo.

Schildgen, Robert. 1988. *Toyohiko Kagawa: Apostle of love and social justice.* Berkeley: Centenary Books. (Translation: ロバート・シルジェン著 2007.『賀川豊彦―愛と社会正義を追い求めた生涯』Tokyo: Shinkyo Shuppansha.)

Sei to seishoku no jinkenmondai shiryō shūsei. 2000-2003.［性と生殖の人権問題資料集成 Collected Materials of Human Rights Problems of Sex and Reproduction］ 35 vols. Tokyo: Fuji Shuppan.

Sugiyama Hiroaki［杉山博昭］. 1998. "Kirisutokyō shakaijigyōka to yūseishisō"［キリスト教社会事業家と優生思想 Christian Social Workers and Eugenic Thought］ in *Kirisutokyō Shakaifukusigaku kenkyū*［基督教社会福祉学研究 Studies of Christian Social Work］ 30, 46-55.

――――. 2003. *Kirisutokyō fukushi jissen no shitekitenkai*［キリスト教福祉実践の史的展開 Historical Development of Christian Welfare Practice］. Okayama: Daigaku Kyoiku Shuppan.

――――. 2010. "Kagawa Toyohiko to yūseishisō"［賀川豊彦と優生思想 Kagawa Toyohiko and Eugenic Thought］ in *Kagawa Toyohiko gakkai ronsō*［賀川豊彦学会論叢 Toyohiko Kagawa Society Review］ 13, 33-48.

Suzuki Masasetsu［鈴木正節］. 1983. *Taishō demokurasii no gunzō*［大正デモクラシーの群像 Persons of Taisho Democracy］, 69-84. Tokyo: Yuzankaku.

Takano Zen'ichi［高野善一］. 1970. *Abe Isoo: Nihon shakaishugi no chichi*［安部磯雄―日本社会主義の父 Abe Isoo: Father of Japanese Socialism］. Tokyo: Abe Isoo Kankōkai.

Tsujino Isao［辻野功］. 1974. *Meiji no kakumeikatachi*［明治の革命家たち Revolutionists of Meiji Period］, 83-122. Tokyo: Yushindo.

―――. 1978. *Meiji shakaishugishiron*［明治社会主義史論 Historical Study of Meiji Socialism］. Kyoto: Hōritsu Bunkasha, 188-220.

Wakagi Chikako［若木千賀子］. 1966. "Abe Isoo shisō keiseiron"［安部磯雄思想形成論 An Inner Analysis of Abe Isoo's Thought］in *Joshi Seigakuin kenkyū kiyō*［女子聖学院研究紀要 Joshi Seigakuin Research Review］3, 1-28.

Yamaizumi Susumu［山泉進］. 1981. "Shakaishugi to hakuai no seishin［社会主義と博愛の精神〈安部磯雄〉Socialism and Spirit of Philanthropy: Abe Isoo］in *Kindai Nihon to Waseda no shisō gunzō*［近代日本と早稲田の思想群像］Waseda Daigaku Shakaikagaku Kenkyūsho Nihon Kindai Shisōbukai ed., 209-233. Tokyo: Waseda Daigaku Shuppanbu.

―――, ed. 2001. *Shakaishugi no tanjō: shakai minshutō hyakunen*［社会主義の誕生―社会民主党百年］Tokyo: Ronsōsha.

―――, ed. 2003. *Heiminsha hyakunen korekushon. Dai 3 kan: Abe Isoo*［平民社百年コレクション 第3巻 安部磯雄 Commoners' Society Century Collection Vol. 3: Abe Isoo］. Tokyo: Ronsosha.

―――, ed. 2008. *Heiminsha no Jidai: Hisen no Genryū*［平民社の時代―非戰の源流 Period of Commoners' Society: A Source of Pacifism］. Tokyo: Ronsosha.

Chapter 4

"Good Wives, Wise Mothers" and "Racial Poisons" in Japan

Karen J. Schaffner

Eugenic thought played a role Japan's process of modernization and civilization. Western ideas about how to deal with social problems and how to improve society were selectively incorporated. One of those ideas came from British physician and journalist, Caleb Williams Saleeby. He maintained that "racial poisons" needed to be eliminated from society to preserve its health and improve its quality. His list included "alcohol, lead, narcotics, and syphilis" (Saleeby 1909, 228). As his idea spread, inherited weakness, tuberculosis, prostitution, criminality, pauperism, and tobacco were added to the list. Some of these also became issues of concern in Japan. In this chapter, the role of women in addressing some of Japan's "racial poisons"[1] will be examined.

Women had been assigned the role of "good wife, wise mother" (*ryōsai kenbo*[2]) (See Uno 1993, 2008). Excluded from participation in political activities by Article 5 of the Public Order and Police Law (*Chian keisatsu-hō*[3]) and relegated to motherhood and the upkeep of the home, women had to find a way to deal with the social problems which threatened them and their families. The forums available to them were magazines and lectures. For any attempt at exerting political influence, they were forced to rely on men to present their petitions to the Diet.

1. Temperance[4]

One of the "racial poisons" identified by eugenic thought that affected women was alcohol. With encouragement and help from American female activists, Japanese women organized the Tokyo Woman's Christian Temperance Union (WCTU *Tokyo Kirisutokyō fujin kyōfū kai*[5]) in 1886. Through lectures and publications and with the cooperation of men of similar persuasion, they made their appeal for abstinence. A lecture meeting held in Tokyo in November 1887 attracted some one thousand participants. Tsuda Sen's[6] lecture, entitled "*Sake no gai*"[7] (The Dangers of Alcohol), outlined the harm which accompanied alcohol consumption—physical and mental

---

1. 人種の毒　2. 良妻賢母　3. 治安警察法　4. 禁酒，断酒
5. 日本キリスト教婦人矯風会　6. 津田仙　7. 「酒の害」

weakness, shortened life span, mental disabilities in children whose mothers who drank—along with crime and its cost to society. In addition to lectures, the WCTU also sponsored recitation contests among young people and exhibitions at expositions (Lublin 2010, 126-148).

Such gatherings helped educate people, but a change in laws had to come from the Diet. The Diet member recruited to present a petition to ban underage drinking was Nemoto Shō,[1] whose wife was also active in the temperance movement (Katō Junji 1999; see also Otsubo 2006). The bill was first presented in the Lower House in 1901, but without success. It was presented every year thereafter until it passed both houses in 1922. The passage of the prohibition law in the United States seemed to provide the impetus for its passage in the House of Peers. The Juvenile Alcohol Prohibition Act (*Miseinensha inshu kinshi-hō*[2]) banned the sale of alcoholic beverages to minors and their use by minors. Parents and guardians were responsible for keeping their offspring from using alcohol.

2. Tobacco

Similarly, the effect of tobacco on young people was addressed by the WCTU. In their exhibits at expositions and in lectures, they sought to educate people about the dangers of smoking. They encouraged the passage of a bill to ban underage smoking. Nemoto Shō, along with four other representatives, presented the petition to the Lower House of the Diet in December 1899, the year after he was elected to the lower house of the Diet. Unlike the bill to prevent minors from drinking liquor, the *Miseinensha kitsuen kinshi-hō*[3] [Law prohibiting the smoking of tobacco by minors] passed both houses the first time it was presented and was put into effect from April 1900. During the discussion of the bill, the argument that helped clinch its passage was that the use of tobacco had a detrimental effect on the health of soldiers. The bill prohibited the use of tobacco by minors under the age of twenty and made those who sold tobacco or smoking paraphernalia to minors liable to a fine. Parents were to exercise parental authority to prevent their children from smoking. They, too, were subject to fines for failure to do so. The passage of this bill was a victory for "wise mothers," who wanted to protect their families from being poisoned by tobacco.

3. Prostitution[4]

Besides working to prohibit the use of alcohol and tobacco, the WCTU also put a

---

1. 根本正　　2. 未成年者飲酒禁止法　　3. 未成年者喫煙禁止法　　4. 売春

strong priority on abolishing public prostitution. Elisabeth Lublin draws attention to three aspects of their efforts: "agitation against Japanese prostitutes overseas, opposition to particular brothel[1] districts, and rescue efforts" (Lublin 2010, 101). The second aspect will be the focus of this section.

One early campaign was instigated in Osaka starting in 1902. The Union drew up a petition urging that brothel areas be moved from the center to the outskirts of town. They provided information for each legislator, conducted lectures, and made their appeal in the media to protect young people and future generations from an impure atmosphere. Despite not being able to raise enough support to combat brothel owners' opposition, members of the Union continued their crusade.

A fire which reached the centrally located Sonezaki pleasure district[2] in July 1909 prompted the Union to make concerted efforts to prevent its reconstruction and have it moved from Osaka's populated area. These efforts included expansion of their support base. The Union was already working with YMCA directors and Protestant ministers to provide relief to the victims of the fire, but their cooperation in collecting signatures for petitions, holding public lectures, and distributing printed information was also acquired. Visits were made to officials to make their pleas and present their signed petitions. Their efforts in rallying support were successful. In September, the governor announced that all brothel licenses would be terminated in April 1910.

This victory inspired movements in other areas, such as Gunma prefecture and Wakayama city. Employing a similar strategy as had been used in Osaka, women and sympathetic men were successful in getting decisions to allow prostitution districts overturned.

In 1911, Tokyo's Yoshiwara[3] district was chosen as the next target. As in Osaka, a fire broke out in the district, quickly spreading in the densely constructed wooden structures and destroying homes, schools, temples, businesses, and brothels. Again wide public support was achieved, and petitions were delivered to officials. But neither the public opinion of Tokyo residents nor the assurance that ridding Tokyo of "its darkest and most inhumane spot" (Lublin 2010, 117) would raise Japan's international assessment was enough to move the Yoshiwara district from its original location.

When the crusade to shut down Yoshiwara ended in defeat, the need for an ongoing movement against brothels and prostitution became apparent. In May 1911 members of the WCTU joined forces with other activists to form the *Kakuseikai*[4] (Purity Society), whose purpose was to "abolish the system of licensed prostitution and promote pure relations between men and women" (Lublin 2010, 117; see Chapter 4 in this volume). These two groups, working together, were able to persuade fifteen prefectural assemblies

1. 売春宿   2. 曾根崎遊郭   3. 吉原   4. 廓清会

to outlaw prostitution by the early 1940s, but nationwide legislation was not enacted until 1957 (Lublin 2010, 118; Nihon Kirisutokyō fujin kyōfūkai 1986, 605-13, 1038).

4. Venereal Disease

A "racial poison" connected with prostitution was venereal disease. In Japanese the expression often used was *karyūbyō*[1] [lit. disease of red light district]. Wives were often infected by their husbands who frequented brothels. Hiratsuka Raichō[2] and members of the *Shin fujin kyōkai*[3] (New Woman Association) began a movement to protect women from the "racial poison" of venereal disease (see Otsubo 1998, Chapter 4; 1999, 2006). Their proposal was that premarital testing for venereal disease be required of men. Hiratsuka had a petition to that effect presented in the December 1919 Diet session. The legislators she recruited encouraged her to justify testing for men only. She appealed to Japan's desire to be counted among the "civilized" countries. While Western countries had acknowledged the impact and spread of venereal disease and had taken legal measures to deal with the problem, Japan had not. She argued that men were more likely to be exposed to disease because of sexual contact outside the home and that the gynecological testing of women was culturally inappropriate. Her assumption was that sexual diseases were largely limited to prostitutes. Her final argument stressed "the protection of housewives and their children would improve the quality of the nation (*kokumin*[4]) and strengthen national power (*kokuryoku*[5]) (Otsubo 2006, 232).

Although the petition was given serious consideration, and the need for legislation to address venereal disease was acknowledged, the bill never went beyond committee discussion due to dissolution of the Diet. However, this initial attempt attracted attention in magazines, in both those for women and men.

A second attempt was made in the summer of the following year. Nemoto Shō was one of the presenters to the committee of the House of Representatives and, in the end, the only supporter of the proposal. Sumiko Otsubo notes that "the primary reason for its rejection was its gendered aspect, requiring only men to submit a medical certificate before marriage" (Otsubo 2006, 235).

Having the door closed to legislative reform, Hiratsuka and her supporters formed a group of women who agreed to refuse marriage to a man with V. D. (*Karyūbyō danshi kyokon dōmei*[6]). There were voices of support and criticism for this move, but the problem of venereal disease continued to be discussed in the media. A new petition requiring women to produce a health certificate on demand and including coverage of common law marriages garnered 2,500 supporting signatories, 1,000 of whom were

1. 花柳病   2. 平塚らいてう   3. 新婦人協会   4. 国民   5. 国力
6. 花柳病男子拒婚同盟

males (Otsubo 2006, 238).

At the end of January 1921 a revised petition was submitted for committee discussion in the Lower House. Rather than having to produce a medical document to prospective brides, men would present a license from a municipal office certifying them to be disease free. Women could be asked to provide a similar document if the prospective husband so desired. An appeal to the eugenic aspects of the proposal—protection of the state and its citizens—was made. Again, the petition did not make it out of the committee, but dissenting members were few. This defeat, as well as the defeat of the petition to revise the Public Order and Police Law, brought an end to the attempt to enact a law to protect women from the "racial poison" of venereal disease.

5. Inherited Weakness[1]

The "racial poison" of inherited weakness was also seen as a threat to women and their families. According to eugenic thought, this threat could be countered by "wise" marriages, eugenic marriages. On June 20, 1933, a eugenics marriage consultation[2] center was opened in Tokyo's Shiraki-ya Department Store by the Japan Society of Race Hygiene[3] (*Minzoku eisei* 2:6, 87-88). Two years later on November 11, the society founded the Eugenics Marriage Popularization Society.[4] Unlike its affiliated society, this one consisted entirely of women. With Nagai Hisomu[5] at the head, all the other officers were women— "professionals, wives of prominent men, and daughters from distinguished families" (Otsubo 1998, 274), including Nagai's wife Hanae.[6]

The Society offered consultation on marriage issues. Visitors could receive counseling in medical matters and hereditary matters. For those who were unable or unwilling to visit the society, information was available in a monthly journal *Yūsei*.[7] In the first issue (March 1936) readers were informed concerning eugenic marriage and concerning their vital role in building the nation of Japan:

> Choosing a spouse of good quality, avoiding one of poor quality, and ensuring the physical and mental fitness of descendants is a source of the well-being of immediate, as well as extended, family in smaller context. It is also the foundation of the betterment of state (*kokka*[8]) and ethnic nation (*minzoku*[9]) in a larger context (Otsubo 1998, 284).

Positive eugenics—encouraging the birth of fit offspring—and negative eugenics—preventing the birth of unfit offspring—were introduced in subsequent issues. Marriage

---

1. 遺伝する薄弱　2. 優生結婚相談所　3. 日本民族衛生学会　4. 優生結婚普及会
5. 永井潜　6. 永井花江　7. 『優生』　8. 国家　9. 民族

to "men who had such 'ethnic national poisons' (*minzokudoku*[1]) as venereal diseases, tuberculosis,[2] leprosy,[3] and drinking problems themselves or in their families" was discouraged (Otsubo 1998, 285). Such weakness could be passed on to children and harm families, as well as the nation. Included in the journal were also news articles and marriage advice columns.

Concluding Remarks

Women in pre-Pacific war Japan were assigned the role of producing, nurturing, and educating the next generation of Japanese. Relegated to activities centered around the home, women had few outlets for changing the society in which they lived. In eugenic thought, women found a cause for which to work. As "good wives and wise mothers," they made efforts to protect themselves and their families from "racial poisons" which could destroy both the family and the nation. These included alcohol, tobacco, venereal disease, prostitution, and inherited weakness. Not included are two which are conspicuous in their absence. One is tuberculosis. Sumiko Otsubo suggests that Hiratsuka Raichō did not pursue this issue to avoid bringing harm to factory women, many of whom were infected with tuberculosis (Otsubo 1998, 154). A second is leprosy. (See Chapter 9.) This, like tuberculosis, was addressed by government agencies and medical doctors. Measures were taken against individuals in the name of protecting the nation.

Not all of the women's attempts were successful in achieving their goals. But, even in defeat, "eugenics empowered women and helped them develop self-esteem, confidence, and consciousness about their bodies, and thereby had a potential to challenge the very ideology which supported social structure of the state" (Otsubo 1998, 33). Although shut out of political participation, women were able to work for the well-being of themselves and their families in ways that went beyond the patriarchal society's definition of "good wives and wise mothers." However, at the same time, eugenic policies of the state put them in a position of being monitored and manipulated. Women were expected to have many children to supply the needs of the state's military. Their health was supervised, and the good of the nation was put before individual choices and freedom.

References

Frühstück, Sabine. 2000. "Managing the Truth of Sex in Imperial Japan." *The Journal of Asian Studies* 59:2, 332-358.

———. 2003. *Colonizing Sex: Sexology and Social Control in Modern Japan*. Berkeley: Uni-

1. 民族毒   2. 結核   3. らい病（ハンセン病）

versity of California Press.

Garon, Sheldon. 1993. "The World's Oldest Debate? Prostitution and the State in Imperial Japan, 1900-1945" in *American Historical Review* 98.3, 710-732.

Hiratsuka Raichō ［平塚らいてう］. 1919. "Gendai katei fujin no nayami" ［現代家庭婦人の悩み Today's domestic women's worry］ in *Shiryō: bosei hogo ronsō*, Kouchi Nobuko, ed. Reprint 1984. Tokyo: Domesu Shuppan.

Itō Hidekichi ［伊藤秀吉］. 1931. *Nihon haishōundōshi* ［日本廃娼運動史 History of the movement to abolish prostitution in Japan］. Reprint 1995. Tokyo: Fuji Shuppan.

Katō Junji ［加藤純二］. 1999~. "Miseinensha inshu/kitsuen kinshi-hō to Nemoto Shō" ［未成年者飲酒・喫煙禁止法と根本正 Law to prevent drinking/smoking by minors］ 〈http://www.geocities.jp/m_kato_clinic/nemo-haikei-1.html〉

———. 1999~ "Leaflet about three laws drafted by Sho Nemoto" 〈http://www.geocities.jp/m_kato_clinic/nemo-leaflet-eng-01.html〉

Lublin, Elizabeth Dorn. 2010. *Reforming Japan: The Women's Christian Temperance Union in the Meiji Period*. Vancouver: University of British Columbia Press.

Molony, Barbara. 1993. "Equality versus Difference: The Japanese Debate over 'Motherhood Protection,' 1915-50" in *Japanese Women Working*, Janet Hunter, ed., 122-148. London: Routledge.

———. 2008. "The Quest for Women's Rights in Turn-of-the Century Japan" in *Gendering Modern Japanese History*, Barbara Molony and Kathleen S. Uno, eds., 463-483. Cambridge, MA: Council on East Asian Studies, Harvard University.

Nihon Kirisutokyō Fujin Kyōfūkai ［日本キリスト教婦人矯風会］. 1913~. *Fujin shimpō* ［婦人新報 Woman's herald］. Reprint 1986. Tokyo: Fuji Shuppan.

———. 1986. *Nihon Kirisutokyō Fujin Kyōfūkai Hyakunenshi* ［日本キリスト教婦人矯風会百年史 One hundred year history of the Japan Woman's Christian Temperance League］. Tokyo: Domesu Shuppan.

Orii, Miyako ［折井美耶子］ and Hiroko Tomida. 2005. "*Shin Fujin Kyōkai* (the Association of New Women) and the Women Who aimed to Change Society" in *Japanese Women: Emerging from Subservience, 1868-1945*, Hiroko Tomida & Gordon Daniels, eds., 232-257. Kent: Global Oriental Ltd.

Ostubo (Sitcawich), Sumiko. 1998. *Eugenics in Imperial Japan: Some Ironies of Modernity, 1883-1945*. Ph.D. dissertation, Ohio State University.

———. 1999. "Feminist Maternal Eugenics in Wartime Japan" in *U.S.-Japan Women's Journal* (English Supplement) 17:39-76.

——— ［大坪寿美子］. 2006. "Toward a Common Eugenic Goal: Christian Social Reformers and the Medical Authorities in Meiji and Taisho Japan" in *Dōtoku to Kagaku no Intāfēsu: Kindaika no Ichisokumen* ［道徳と科学のインターフェース：近代化の一側面 The Interface of Morality and Science] *Kōnan Daigaku Sōgōkenkyūjo sōsho* ［申南大学総合研究所叢書］ 86 (April), 43-86.

———. 2008. "Engendering Eugenics: Japanese Feminists and Marriage Restriction Legislation (1919-1922)" in *Gendering Modern Japanese History*, Barbara Molony and Kathleen S. Uno, eds., 225-247. Cambridge, MA: Council on East Asian Studies, Harvard University.

Robertson, Jennifer. 2005. "Biopower: Blood, Kinship, and Eugenic Marriage" in *A Companion to the Anthropology of Japan*, Jennifer Robertson, ed., 329-354. Malden, MA: Blackwell Publishing.

———. 2012. "Eugenics in Japan: Sanguinous Repair" in *The Oxford Handbook of the History of Eugenics*, Alison Bashford and Philippa Levine, eds., 430-448. New York: Oxford University Press.

Saleeby, Caleb Williams. 1909. "The Obstacles to Eugenics" in *Sociological Review* 2:3 (July) 228-240.

Tsuda Sen ［津田仙］. 1889. *Sake no gai* ［酒の害 The Dangers of Alcohol］. Gakunōsha zasshikyoku.

Uno, Kathleen S. 1993. "The Death of 'Good Wife, Wise Mother'?" in *Postwar Japan as History*, Andrew Gordon, ed., 293-322. Berkley: University of California Press.

———. 2008. "Women, Empire, and War: Transmutations of 'Good Wife, Wise Mother' before 1931" in *Gendering Modern Japanese History*, Barbara Molony and Kathleen S. Uno, eds., 493-513. Cambridge, MA: Council on East Asian Studies, Harvard University.

Part II

Japanese Eugenics Connections

Chapter 5   *Japan-U.S. Eugenics Connections*

Karen J. Schaffner

At the First International Eugenics Congress[1] held in London (1912), delegates from around the world gathered to hear papers presented on the relationship of eugenics to biology, education, and sociology. How to increase the reproduction of the "fit" and reduce that of the "unfit" was an often discussed topic. After this congress, the center of eugenics shifted to the United States, where a number of associations, publications, and foundations based on eugenic ideas were established, often funded by wealthy philanthropists. Their publications and activities provided information, education, and resources for the eugenics movement. Each sought to spread eugenic ideas and policies not only in the United States, but around the world.

This chapter will focus on the leaders of four American eugenic organizations and their connections with Japan: the Eugenics Record Office,[2] the American Eugenics Society[3], the Human Betterment Foundation, and the American Birth Control League. Translations of publications, contact with American eugenicists, and correspondence with them provide insight into the role American eugenics played in Japan.

1. Eugenics Record Office (ERO)

Established in 1910 in Cold Spring Harbor, Long Island, New York, adjacent to the Carnegie Institute sponsored Station for Experimental Evolution,[4] the Eugenics Record Office served as a "meeting place for eugenicists, a repository for eugenic records, a clearinghouse for eugenic information and propaganda, a platform from which popular eugenic campaigns could be launched, and a home for several eugenical publications" (Allen 1986, 302). The office was under the direction of Charles B. Davenport,[5] with Harry H. Laughlin[6] as assistant director. The ERO devised a form for gathering family pedigree[7] information, trained field workers to gather information, and published family studies and, from 1916, the periodical *Eugenical News*.[8] The ERO focused its efforts on campaigning for sterilizing "unfit" citizens and restricting "unfit" immigrants.

1. 第1回国際優生学会議   2. 優生記録局   3. アメリカ優生協会   4. 実験進化研究所
5. チャールズ・B. ダヴェンポート   6. ハリー・H. ロフリン   7. 家系図
8. 『優生学ニュース』

In Davenport's correspondence, deposited at the American Philosophical Society Library, are letters to and from several Japanese. Scientists studying in America, such as Tokyo Imperial University professor Ishikawa Chiyomatsu,[1] visited Davenport at Cold Spring Harbor. Others, like Abe Fumio,[2,*1] were aware of Davenport's research and requested further information from him. Still others, such as Kyoto Imperial University professor Komai Taku,[3] who had met him at the Third International Eugenics Congress, subscribed to ERO publications, and sent Davenport articles for publication in American eugenics journals.

Davenport's studies of animal breeding formed the basis of his study of heritable traits in humans. *Heredity in Relation to Eugenics* (1911) reflects his stance on the aims of eugenics and the importance of good breeding.

> The general program of the eugenist [sic] is clear—it is to improve the race by inducing young people to make a more reasonable selection of marriage mates; to fall in love intelligently. It also includes the control by the state of the propagation of the mentally incompetent (Davenport 1911, 4).

Davenport also emphasized the genetic nature of race, the dangers of interracial breeding, and the genetic nature of defective traits such as feeblemindedness, epilepsy, and insanity.

In 1914, Davenport's *Heredity in Relation to Eugenics* was selected for translation by the Greater Japan Civilization Society,[4] begun in 1908 after Japan's victory in the Russo-Japanese War. The purpose of the society was to search for new knowledge, to provide educational nourishment for a new era, and to gauge the harmonious blending of Eastern and Western civilization. With the publication of some 200 books, the society introduced many European and American scholars to Japan.

Gotō Ryūkichi,[5] a medical journalist in the Kansai area and founder of the Japan Eugenics Society,[6] read Davenport's book [*Jinshu kairyōgaku*[7]] and worked to promote eugenics among Japanese (see Ostubo 1998, Chapter 5). In 1924, he started a monthly magazine, *Yūzenikkusu*[8] [Eugenics, from 1925 *Yūseigaku*[9]]. Having neither a governmental nor an academic position, Gotō struggled to broaden his readership and keep his magazine in the black. Although he had sympathizers among academicians, he received only token support and had to depend heavily on advertising sales. In a letter dated June 15, 1924, Gotō solicited help from Davenport to solve his dilemma.

> Wonld [sic] yon [sic] be kind enough to let us take the liberty of writing to

1. 石川千代松   2. 阿部文夫   3. 駒井卓   4. 大日本文明協会   5. 後藤竜吉
6. 日本優生学会   7.『人種改良学』   8.『ユーゼニックス』   9.『優生学』

yon [sic], hoping sincerely your help and encouragement in a llrespects [sic], as we have little experience in this line of magazine business? (*Yūseigaku* 2:2 [1925], 6).

Davenport's prompt reply on July 2 provided the help and encouragement Gotō sought:

> We should be glad to assist you in any way that we can. In response to your request, we are sending you a paper by Dr. Laughlin on the organization of the Eugenics Record Office, an account of the Department of Genetics which includes the Eugenics Record Office. We are also sending you a number of our schedules.
> We should be glad in return to receive what you have published" (*Yūseigaku* 2: 3 [1925], 6).

Thus the connection was established, and translations of articles from the ERO and the *Eugenical News* began to appear in Gotō's magazine. His readers were able to read about topics such as the work of the ERO, hereditary feeblemindedness and mental disorders, and the racial traits of athletes. "Schedules" from the ERO were used to record family traits and the results used to develop pedigree charts which also appeared in the magazine. Information about eugenics in Japan was also sent to the ERO and included in the *Eugenical News*.

2. The American Eugenics Society (AES)

One of the members of Gotō's Japan Eugenics Society was Kaneko Tadakazu,[1] a natural science teacher at the Tokyo First Higher School for Girls. He was listed on the American Eugenics Society membership list beginning in 1930 and was a contact for a 1931 lecture tour by Roswell Hill Johnson,[2] conducted under the auspices of the AES.

Johnson had studied under Charles Davenport and had done research at the Station for Experimental Evolution. Afterwards at the University of Pittsburgh, he organized one of America's first eugenics and social hygiene courses. He was a founding member of the AES and held various roles, including president and secretary/treasurer.

Johnson became known in Japan when his book *Applied Eugenics*,[3] coauthored with Paul B. Popenoe[4] (editor for the American Breeders Association's[5] *Journal of Heredity*[6]), was selected for the Greater Japan Civilization Society's collection in 1922. The book, originally published in 1918, was widely used as a text for American college eugenics classes as well as for a popular audience.

1. 金子直一　2. ロズウェル・ヒル・ジョンソン　3. 『応用優生学』
4. ポール・B. ポペノー　5. アメリカ育種家協会　6. 『遺伝ジャーナル』

During a 1928 stopover in Japan, Johnson's interest in Japan's social problems was aroused. He was confident eugenics held the solutions to those problems. When it was reported that "an imperial Commission had been organized in Japan for a study of eugenical principles and legislation with a view to setting up a eugenics program in that country" (*Eugenics* 2:3, 29), Johnson, who was then serving as secretary of the society, was authorized to offer the society's help and cooperation to the newly established commission. Leon Whitney, then president of the society, noted that

> Johnson returned with the impression that the Japanese are as keenly alive to the subject as are the people of almost any other country.... Sterilization and race betterment are indeed becoming ideas among all enlightened nations to-day" (Whitney, 1934, 139).

Details of the 1931 lecture trip were published in the November 1931 issue of *Eugenical News* (16:11, 195) and a more extensive report sent to Ezra S. Gosney of the Human Betterment Foundation[1] (Johnson 1934a). Johnson gained firsthand information about eugenics in Japan from visits to various institutions, including the Tokyo Joint Prefectural Sanatorium[2] and the Imperial Leprosarium on the Inland Sea,[3] a mental hospital, a penitentiary, a reformatory, and Kawada's School for the Feebleminded on Ōshima Island.[4]

During his stay in Japan, he delivered 29 lectures in 23 cities to some 1,190 persons. The Public Health Division of the Home Office[5] made the arrangements for most of the venues, including Sapporo, Asahikawa, Niigata, Nagano, Nagoya, Kyoto, Osaka, Kobe, Hiroshima, Fukuoka, Kumamoto, and Nagasaki. Kaneko made arrangements for lectures at the Kanda YMCA in Tokyo, in Hirosaki, and in Morioka.

Available information indicates that some of Johnson's lectures dealt with birth control. The title of the YMCA lecture was "The Problems of Birth Control from a Eugenics Perspective."[6] Johnson's address to the First American Birth Control Conference of 1921 provides insight into his position on birth control.

> Our most pressing problem is to increase the birth rate from the superior and to decrease from the inferior.... The reasons which impel the women who clamor for information on Birth Control are poor health, insufficient time for proper recovery since birth of last child, and above all, the financial inability to support the additional children.... Birth control is not birth repression, but truly birth control—that is more births from superior and less from inferior (Johnson 1921).

---

1. 人間改良財団   2. 国立ハンセン病療養所   3. 長島愛生園   4. 大島の藤倉学園
5. 内務省衛生局   6. 「優生学上より見たる産児制限の諸問題」

A second topic of Johnson's lectures was sterilization.[1] In August 1931, he lectured about the legal aspects of sterilization to the Japan Association of Mental Hygiene.[2] For Johnson, sterilization was one way of limiting the reproduction of the "unfit," but not a substitute for other methods, such as segregation,[3] contraception,[4] and marriage licensing.[5] By removing the danger of reproduction, sterilization was best suited for cases where the person did not require institutionalization, or where release of patients could free space for others who did.

Johnson felt that "the eugenic movement will proceed faster in Japan than elsewhere in the Orient" because of its "strong government, a strong social spirit that is less individualistic than in the West, lack of any serious obstacle from either equalitarian or religious ideals and the existence of strong racial pride" (Johnson 1934b, 193). He also predicted that "Japan within the next generation or two will be one of the world's leaders in the promotion of a eugenic population policy" (Popenoe 1933, 369). While in Japan, he emphasized sterilization of the feebleminded, insane, and alcoholics to be of greater value for the improvement of society (Johnson 1934b, 191).

3. Human Betterment Foundation (HBF)

Sterilization was the focus of research for the Human Betterment Foundation, a third American eugenics organization with Japanese connections. The HBF was founded in Pasadena, California and formally incorporated in 1928. Johnson's report of his trip to Japan was addressed to its founder—businessman and philanthropist Ezra Seymour Gosney.[6] According to the HBF charter, its purpose was "the advancement and betterment of human life, character and citizenship," not accomplished by relief work or charitable activities, but by education, making the need for relief work unnecessary (HBF 1928). Through scientific investigation, the foundation proposed to provide Americans with advice concerning how to better the human family by sterilizing the unfit.

In the spring of 1926 with Paul B. Popenoe as research coordinator, HBF began gathering data from five state institutions doing sterilization operations for eugenic purposes. The results were published in *Sterilization for Human Betterment: A Summary of Results of 6,000 Operations in California, 1909-1929* and in *Twenty-eight Years of Sterilization in California*. These studies set out to show the effectiveness of sterilization in controlling the multiplication of the feebleminded and the reproduction of the mentally handicapped. From the first sterilization law passed in Indiana in 1907 until 1917, 1,422 operations were performed nationwide—seventy per cent of which were in California. Throughout the 1930s, California continued to have the largest number of surgeries.

1. 断種 2. 日本精神衛生協会 3. 隔離 4. 避妊 5. 結婚許可証の使用
6. エズラ・シーモア・ガスニー

From 1930 to 1944, this number totaled nearly 11,000. In 1941, the year before Gosney's death and the dissolution of the foundation, twenty-nine states had sterilization laws, and the total number of operations nationwide was 38,087 (Reilly, 1991, 96-100).

Gosney's efforts were not limited to America. He also made contacts with eugenicists in Japan. Correspondence with Japanese[*2] found in Gosney's papers centers on Waseda University professor, Christian socialist, and politician Abe Isoo[1] (see Chapter 4). Abe met Gosney when he traveled to the United States in 1929. He saw the work of the HBF firsthand at a California institution for the "feebleminded," where he observed young men and women of limited mental ability being sterilized with their parents' permission or even at their request. He became convinced that Japan, too, needed eugenic sterilization. Abe translated Gosney's and Popenoe's *Sterilization for Human Betterment*,[2] which was published in 1930 by the Greater Japan Civilization Society. He also used materials from HBF pamphlets in essays he wrote for other magazines.

Nagai Hisomu,[3] who would later draft a sterilization law for Japan, also introduced Gosney in the journal of the Japan Society of Race Hygiene [*Nihon Minzoku Eisei Gakkai*].[4] The June 1934 edition was dedicated to Gosney and the topic of sterilization. This was the same year that efforts began to introduce sterilization legislation in the Japanese Imperial Diet. Although early attempts were unsuccessful, subsequent ones were made until it was passed in 1940.

Whenever the introduction of sterilization legislation in the Japanese Parliament was reported in the American press, Gosney wrote to inquire about the bill's origin and probability of its passage, offering to offer help to get out the real facts concerning sterilization. In a December 1936 letter to Abe, he asked about reported plans to submit a "bill for sterilization of the insane,[5] epileptics,[6] confirmed alcoholics,[7] and persons of known criminal tendencies"[8] in the next meeting of Parliament. He notes, "Such a law in Japan, conservatively and humanly administered would do much for the betterment of the human family not only in Japan but in all civilized countries." Abe's reply expressed hope that his party would gain a majority and be able to pass the legislation. He also commented that the nearly fifty thousand lepers[9] in Japan illustrated the necessity of such legislation. Gosney's September letter sought confirmation of the targeted group.

> I suppose you intend to include sterilization of selected parties, who are feebleminded—though you do not say so. The sterilization of the feebleminded in California has been more universally approved than the sterilization of any other class of defectives (Gosney 1937).

1. 安部磯雄　2. 『不妊結婚と人間改造』　3. 永井潜　4. 日本民族衛生学会
5. 精神病患者　6. てんかん患者　7. 筋金入りのアルコール中毒者
8. 既知の犯罪性のある者　9. らい患者（ハンセン病患者）

This kind of exchange was repeated again in 1939—Gosney emphasizing the sterilization of the feebleminded and Abe that of Hansen's disease patients.

With the formation of a eugenics division within the Ministry of Health and Welfare[1] and the help of bureaucrats, a bill was submitted to the Diet and passed both houses in 1940 to become the "National Eugenic Law."[2] This bill sought to prevent an increase of genetically inferior descendants and at the same time to increase the number of healthy descendants. Abortion was strictly restricted. Due to opposition from various groups, the small number of those meeting the necessary requirements in institutions, as well as the need to "be fruitful and multiply"[3] to provide soldiers for the war, the number of those sterilized under the law was limited—454 from 1941 to 1945 (Takeda 2005, 205).

4. American Birth Control League (Planned Parenthood Federation of America[4] 1942)

The beginning of the birth control movement in Japan was connected to Margaret Sanger.[5*3] Her ideas and methods were seen as a possible answer to Japan's population problems after World War I. Baroness Ishimoto Shidzue[6] met Sanger in 1920 in New York and afterwards was determined to introduce birth control ideas in Japan. Though raised in quite different environments, both women had seen the plight of impoverished women for whom frequent and unwanted pregnancies were a drain on their physical strength and their financial ability to care for their children. In March 1922, when Sanger came to visit and lecture, the controversy surrounding her and her arrival provided publicity and name recognition for birth control in Japan.

In July 1922, the Baron and Baroness Ishimoto started the Japan Birth Control Study Society[7] which included others, such as social reformer Abe Isoo, labor activist Katō Kanjū,[8] and feminist Yamakawa Kikue.[9] They gathered to share ideas and to garner support for an organization to promote birth control. Biology professor Yamamoto Senji,[10] who had translated some of Sanger's talks and pamphlets, set up a study group in the Kansai area the following year. With medical doctor Majima Kan,[11*4] he published the *Birth Control Monthly*, providing information primarily to workers.

Government tolerance for the promotion of birth control was mixed. At the 6th International Neo-Malthusian and Birth Control Conference in 1925 held in New York, Abe reported that, while free to speak or write theoretically and send information through the mail, birth control advocates had to have government approval for public speeches and publications concerning birth control (Abe 1925). The planned attempt to gain

1. 厚生省予防局衛生課   2. 国民優生法   3. 「産めよ殖やせよ」
4. アメリカ産児制限同盟・アメリカ家族計画連盟   5. マーガレット・サンガー
6. 石本静枝   7. 日本産児調節研究会   8. 加藤勘十   9. 山川菊枝   10. 山本宣治
11. 馬島僩

governmental support for relaxing anti-abortion laws and allowing contraceptives did not materialize. Yamamoto, who had been elected to the Diet in 1928, was supposed to present the petition to the Lower House in 1929. However, for reasons not related to his support of birth control, he was killed by a right-wing assassin before his presentation.

As mobilization for war accelerated, the government became less tolerant of activities to limit families. Majima was imprisoned for eight months in 1935 for performing illegal abortion. In December of 1937, Ishimoto spent two weeks in jail where she was interrogated about birth control activity and her support of Katō. In January 1938, the government ordered her to close her clinic and to cease all activities to propagate birth control. Medical doctor Ōta Tenrei[1] was also arrested and forced to discontinue his activities.

In postwar Japan, interest in birth control increased due to population growth from the return of repatriates and a rise in the birthrate, as well as a rise in the number of abortions. The occupation government steered clear of the birth control issue, saying it was a matter for the Japanese to decide. Sanger's organization, now called the Planned Parenthood Federation (PPF), wanted to provide assistance, but was given no official recognition. One member of the PPF was especially interested in supporting the cause in Japan. Clarence Gamble,[2] grandson and one of the heirs of the Proctor and Gamble fortune, had used his inheritance to finance birth control activities in the U. S. and around the world. At the end of the occupation, he began making "anonymous" contributions to Katō Shidzue and provided funding to Koya Yoshio[3] for the translation of pamphlets and research projects starting in 1949.

After Majima presented MacArthur a petition signed by some 3,000 Japanese people (Sanger 1953), Margaret Sanger was able to get permission to visit Japan. During her 1952 trip, Margaret Sanger spoke against abortion and for population control. In 1954, she was invited to address a Diet committee and spoke on the topic "Population Problems and Family Planning."[4] The same year Koya Yoshio was made head of the National Institute of Public Health.[5] He had not been supportive of the birth control movement during the war and was not readily accepted by others who had been active in the prewar years.*5

The birth control movement in Japan was splintered into regional efforts with infighting concerning leadership and the proper course of action. After the International Planned Parenthood Federation (IPPF) was organized in 1952, Sanger wrote Koya, Majima, and Katō urging them to present a united front, even if it only existed on paper, so that Japan could become a member (Sanger 1953). Gamble also made efforts to encourage them to cooperate. They, along with others, pulled together, joined the IPPF,

1. 太田典礼　2. クラレンス・ギャンブル　3. 古屋芳雄　4. 「人口問題と家族計画」
5. 国立公衆衛生院

and hosted the 5th International Congress of the IPPF (October, 24-25 1955) in Tokyo.

Concluding Remarks

American eugenics organizations provided information and encouragement in various aspects of eugenics and eugenic policies. Davenport's contribution emphasized genetics and heredity and came largely from publications which were translated into Japanese. He also provided encouragement to researchers who studied in America and to Gotō for his journal. But at the same time, both he and Laughlin were involved in efforts to restrict the immigration of Japanese to America.

Roswell Johnson, on the other hand, brought his sociological view of eugenics to Japan. Unlike Davenport, he pushed for practical policies, such as birth control, segregation,[1] and sterilization, which would, in his way of thinking, improve society. Unlike other American eugenicists who purported racial superiority, Johnson found much to be admired in the Japanese and considered them to be "superior" in many aspects (Johnson 1932).

Gosney provided information on sterilization. His contact and correspondence with Abe show his interest in seeing a sterilization law being passed in Japan. He was respected by Japanese because of the use of his personal funds to set up the HBF.

Sanger looked at birth control from a feminist standpoint, but she and Gamble both were interested in reducing the birth of "unfit." Sanger contributed to the birth control movement in Japan not only with information, but also her "presence." The media's interest in her visits to Japan gave the movement a boost. Gamble, on the other hand, provided funds—not always without strings attached—to further the cause of birth control in postwar Japan.

There was not a wholesale acceptance of what the United States had to offer to Japanese supporters of eugenics. They took the information and selected what fit Japan's situation and needs. Sometimes policies developed in a very different direction than American ones, targeting very different groups of people.

Notes

*1 In correspondence with Davenport, Abe Ayao wrote his first name as "Fumio," an alternate reading of the Japanese characters and presumably easier to understand.

*2 Besides Abe, Gosney had infrequent correspondence with others such as Tokyo Imperial University psychiatric clinic doctor Muramatsu Tsuneo,[2] Kyoto Imperial University psychiatric clinic doctor Mitsuda Hisatoshi,[3] and Kanazawa Medical College doctor Koya Yoshio.

1. 隔離　　2. 村松常雄　　3. 満田久敏

*3 Birth control had already been a topic of discussion among feminists from 1915-1917 in the magazine *Seitō*[1] [Bluestockings]. (See Bardsley 2007, 59ff.)

*4 Instead of Yutaka, Majima used "Kan," the alternate reading of his name, in correspondence with Sanger.

*5 For more about Koya's activities and remarks during the war see Chung 2002, 148-152. Chung has given his surname as "Furuya," which can be an alternate reading of the Japanese characters [古屋].

References

Abe Isoo [安部磯雄]. 1925. "The Birth Control Movement in Japan" in *The Birth Control Review* 9:4 (April), 102, 125-126.

Allen, Garland E. 1986. "The Eugenics Record Office at Cold Spring Harbor, 1920-1940: An Essay in Institutional History" in *Science, Race, and Ethnicity: Readings from Isis and Osiris*, John P. Jackson, Jr., ed., 301-340. Chicago: University of Chicago Press.

American Eugenics Society. 1929. "News and Notes," *Eugenics* 2:3, 29.

Bardsley, Jan. 2007. *The Bluestockings of Japan: New Woman Essays and Fiction from Seitō 1911-16*. Ann Arbor, MI: University of Michigan.

Blacker, C. P. 1956. "Japan's Population Problem" in *The Eugenics Review* 48:1 (Apr.), 31-39.

———. 1963. "Dr. Yoshio Koya: A Memorable Story" in *The Eugenics Review* 55:3 (Oct.), 153-157.

Chung, Juliette Yuehtsen. 2002. *Struggle for National Survival: Eugenics in Sino-Japanese Contexts, 1896-1945*. New York: Routledge.

Davenport, Charles B. 1911. *Heredity in Relation to Eugenics*. New York: Henry Holt and Company.

———. 1914. *Jinshu kairyōgaku* [人種改良学 Study of race betterment] Nakaseko Rokurō [中瀬古六郎] and Yoshimura Daijirō [吉村大次郎] trans. Tokyo: Dainippon Bunmei Kyōkai.

Frühstück, Sabine. 2003. *Colonizing Sex: Sexology and Social Control in Modern Japan*. Berkeley: University of California Press.

Gosney, Ezra S. and Paul Popenoe. 1929. *Sterilization for Human Betterment: A Summary of Results of 6,000 Operations in California, 1909-1929*. New York: Macmillan.

———. 1930. *Funinkekkon to Ningenkaizō* [不妊結婚と人間改造 Barren Marriage and Human Betterment], Abe Isoo, trans. Tokyo: Dainippon Bunmei Kyokai.

———. 1937. "Letter to Isoo Abe, Sept. 10" Box 8, File 3 in E. S. Gosney Papers and Records of the Human Betterment Foundation, 1880-1945. Archives, California Institute of Technology.

Hopper, Helen M. 1996. *A New Woman of Japan: A Political Biography of Kato Shidzue*. Boulder, CO: Westview Press.

Human Betterment Foundation. 1928. "Articles of Incorporation" in E. S. Gosney Papers and

---

1. 『青鞜』

Records of the Human Betterment Foundation, Box 2, File 10. Archives, California Institute of Technology.

Johnson, Roswell Hill. 1921. "Eugenic Aspect of Birth Control" in *Birth Control: what it is, how it works, what it will do; The Proceedings of the First American Birth Control Conference*, 56-58. New York: The Birth Control Review.

———. 1930. "Sterilization: Its Legality, Need" in *Eugenics* 3:5, 180.

———. 1934a. "Report of Eugenic Lecture-Conference trip of Roswell H. Johnson to Japan in 1931 with suggestions to any future lecturer" in E. S. Gosney Papers, Box 24, File 5. Archives, California Institute of Technology.

———. 1934b. *International Eugenics*. Ph. D. dissertation, University of Pittsburgh.

Kato, Shidzue. 1935. *Facing Two Ways: The Story of My Life*. New York: Farrar & Rinehart.

Koya Yoshio. 1963. *Pioneering in Family Planning: A Collection of Papers on the Family Planning and Programs and Research Conducted in Japan*. Tokyo: Japan Medical Publishers.

Nagai Hisomu［永井潜］. 1934. "Jinrui Kaizō Zaidan to sono Sōritsusha Gasunē"［人類改善財団とその創立者ガスネー Human Betterment Foundation and its Founder Gosney］ in *Minzoku Eisei*［民族衛生 Racial Hygiene］3:4-5 (June), 72-78.

Nihon Yūseigakkai［日本優生学会］. 1924-1933. *Yūseigaku*［優生学 Eugenics］. Reprint 2013. Tokyo: Fuji Shuppan.

Ostubo (Sitcawich), Sumiko. 1998. *Eugenics in Imperial Japan: Some Ironies of Modernity, 1883-1945*. Ph.D. dissertation, Ohio State University.

Popenoe, Paul B. and Roswell Hill Johnson. 1918, 1933. *Applied Eugenics*. New York: MacMillan Co.

———. 1922. *Ōyō Yūseigaku*［應用優生學 Applied Eugenics］, Terunuma Tetsunosuke, trans. Tokyo: Dainippon Bunmei Kyokai.

———. 1929. *Ōyō Yūseigaku*［応用優生学 Applied Eugenics］, Hara Sumitsugu［原澄次］, trans. Kyoto: Bunrikaku Shobō.

Reilly, Philip R. 1991. *The Surgical Solution: A History of Involuntary Sterilization in the United States*. Baltimore: John Hopkins University Press.

Sanger, Margaret. 1952-1953. "Letter to Shidzue Kato, Jan. 20, 1952"; "Letter to Yoshio Koya, January 27, 1953"; "Letter to Dr. Kan Majima, Feb. 4, 1953" in Margaret Sanger Papers: Documents from the Sophia Smith Collection.

Schaffner, Karen. 2013. "Nichibei Yūseigaku no Rentai no ichi rei—Rosweru Hiru Jonson—［日米優生学の連帯の一例—ロスウェル・ヒル・ジョンソン— An Example of Japanese and American Eugenics Connections: Roswell Hill Johnson" in *Seimei no rinri 3: Yūsei seisaku no keifu*［生命の倫理3—優生政策の系譜 Ethics of Life 3: The genealogy of eugenic policies］, Yamazaki Kiyoko, ed., 161-191. Fukuoka: Kyushu Daigaku Shuppankai.

———. 2013. "Ningen kairyō no tame no yūseigakuteki danshu—Amerika yūseigaku, Nichi Doku to no rentai—"［人間改良のための優生学的断種—アメリカ優生学，日独との連帯— Eugenic Sterilization for Human Betterment: American eugenics and Japan/Germany Connections］ in *Seimei no rinri 3: Yūsei seisaku no keifu* ［生命の倫理 3—優生政策の系譜 Ethics of Life 3: The genealogy of eugenic policies］, Yamazaki Kiyoko, ed., 55-82. Fukuoka: Kyushu Daigaku Shuppankai.

Takeda Hiroko. 2005. *The Political Economy of Reproduction in Japan: Between Nation-State and Everyday Life.* London: Routledge Curzon.

Takeuchi-Demirci, Aiko. 2011. "The Color of Democracy: A Japanese Public Health Official's Reconnaissance Trip to the U. S. South" in *2010 Southern Spaces series.* 〈https://southernspaces.org/2011/color-democracy-japanese-public-health-officials-reconnaissance-trip-us-south〉

Tipton, Elise. 1997. "Ishimoto Shidzue: the Margaret Sanger of Japan" in *Women's History Review* 6:3, 337-355.

Tokyo Asahi Shimbun ［東京朝日新聞］. 1931. "Gakusha Nihon wo Kōenryokō ［学者日本を講演旅行 Scholar Makes Japan Lecture Trip］ in *Asahi Shimbun* July 19, G3.

Toyoda Maho (豊田真穂). 2010. "Sengo Nihon no Bāsu Kontorōru Undō to Kurarensu Gyamburu" ［戦後日本のバースコントロール運動とクラレンス・ギャンブル Postwar Japan's Birth Control Movement and Clarence Gamble］ in *Jendā Rekishigaku* ［ジェンダー歴史学 The Study of Gender History］ 6, 55-70.

——. 2012. "American Fears in Post-war Japan: Motivations behind Suspending and Promoting Birth Control" in *Synaesthesia Journal* 1:3 (Summer), 91-99.

Whitney, Leon. 1934. *The Case for Sterilization.* New York: Frederick A. Stokes Co. 〈http://openlibrary.org/b/OL7242963M/case_for_sterilization〉

Chapter 6 — *Nazi Sterilization Law and Japan*

Kawashima Sachio

1. Social Problems as the Historical Background of Eugenics

Under the influence of Charles Darwin's[1] evolution and Francis Galton's[2] eugenics in the period of imperialism, social Darwinism[3] spread rapidly among the Western nations. It emphasized the struggle for existence,[4] the law of the jungle, survival of the fittest,[5] and natural selection.[6] German intellectuals were also enamored by eugenic racism, which aimed at increasing the healthy and fit and diminishing the weak and unfit in order to develop and strengthen the nation, race, and state. In the 1850s rapid capitalistic industrialization came to Germany. Social problems, such as bad labor conditions, poor sanitation, diseases, housing shortages, increase in orphans, prostitution, etc., were an embarrassment to the common people.

In 1871 the German Empire was formed under the leadership of Otto von Bismarck as Chancellor. He promoted social legislation to solve social problems, especially social insurance, which was the most progressive in the world at that time. After World War I,[7] under the influence of the Catholic teaching of the principle of "subsidiarity,"[8]*1 the German Weimar Republic began to support civil and religious social work, such as the Inner Mission[9] of the Protestant Church and Caritas[10] of the Catholic Church. Thus the way to a welfare state was prepared, and, at the same time, the cost of welfare and medical treatment increased. These financial burdens, coupled with an increasing military budget, brought the state to a financial crisis in which eugenics began to attract the attention of intellectuals as a solution for social problems.*2

2. Sterilization[11] as a Means of Negative Eugenics

At first, German eugenicists propagated positive eugenics to increase the fit, but did not see very good results. Therefore, they turned their interest to negative eugenics, and were committed to sterilization as a good means of preventing the rapid increase of the

1. チャールズ ダウィン 2. フランシス ゴルトン 3. 社会ダーウィニズム
4. 生存競争 5. 適者生存 6. 自然選択 7. 第一次世界大戦 8. 補完性原理
9. 内国伝道 10. カリタス 11. 断種（不妊手術，優生手術）

disabled and the insane.

The first sterilization legislation was passed in 1907 in Indiana in the United States. This was followed by sterilization laws in some thirty additional American states. In Germany as well, eugenicists appeared who insisted on sterilization legislation. In 1889, psychiatrist and criminologist Paul Näcke[1] proposed sterilization of sexual offenders, and in 1903 psychiatrist Ernst Rüdin[2] supported the sterilization of alcoholics. One reason for these proposals was the economic situation. Otto Juliusburger[3] proposed a compulsory measure: "Think how much money is paid for criminals and insane in sanatoriums, prisons, special education facilities, and mental hospitals" (Juliusburger 1912, 6f ; Thomann 1985, 133).

A famous eugenicist in Germany was physician Alfred Ploetz,[4] who coined the German term—"Rassenhygiene" (race hygiene)[5]—for eugenics. In 1904 he established the eugenic magazine *Archiv für Rassen- und Gesellschaftsbiologie*[6] [Archive for Racial and Social Biology] and in 1905 founded the German Society for Race Hygiene.[7] In 1912 he attended the First International Eugenics Congress[8] in London (Engs, 180f). German eugenicists were influenced by foreigners, especially Americans, through international exchange, correspondence, and books like Géza von Hoffmann's[9] 1913 *Die Rassenhygiene in den Vereinigten Staaten von Nordamerika*[10] [Racial Hygiene in the United States of North America] (Kühl 1994, 16f).

Germany's defeat in World War I changed the eugenic situation. People, especially the intellectuals, felt completely frustrated and began to oppose spending money on welfare and relief facilities, which seemed useless to them. The 1920 book of jurist Karl Binding[11] and psychiatrist Alfred Hoche,[12] *Freigabe der Vernichtung lebensunwerten Lebens*[13] [Release of Extermination of Lives Not Worth Living], defined the lives of so-called idiots "not worthy of life" and suggested that killing them did not fall under the crime of murder from the viewpoints of jurisprudence, medicine, and economy. It called forth no little response, positive and negative, among intellectuals. This book was not regarded as a eugenic one, but it seemed to be a sort of preliminary academic work for legislating the sterilization and the then secret Euthanasia Action[14] of Nazi Germany (Nowak 1984, 48-62).

3. Physician Boeters' Activities for Legislating Sterilization

Medical doctor Gustav Boeters[15] in Zwickau, Saxony is representative of those who publicized the results of sterilization among the public. He not only performed operations, but in 1925 also sent a draft law to the Republic and Saxon state government

1. パウル・ネッケ　　2. エルンスト・リューディン　　3. オットー・ユリウスブルガー
4. アルフレート・プレッツ　　5. 民族（人種）衛生　　6. 『民族・社会生物学雑誌』
7. ドイツ民族衛生協会　　8. 第1回国際優生学会議　　9. ゲーツァ・フォン・ホフマン
10. 『北米合衆国の民族衛生』　　11. カール・ビンディング　　12. アルフレート・ホーヘ
13. 『生きるに値しない生命の抹殺の解禁』　　14. 安楽死作戦　　15. グスタフ・ベータース

for the sterilization of the "feebleminded." It regulated the compulsory sterilization of the congenital blind, deaf and dumb, epileptics, the mentally ill, idiots, the feebleminded, alcoholics, vagabonds, gypsies, etc. His proposal was rejected because its scientific grounds seemed to be too weak to justify sterilization (See Lex Zwickaw 1925 ; Thomann 1985, 136-138 and 181).

4. Prussian Sterilization Draft Bill

The Great Depression,[1] which began with the collapse of the New York stock market, hit Germany severely, and its politics, economy, and society fell into a critical situation. The greatest German state, Prussia, tried then to legislate sterilization as an economic measure. According to the principles on which the Health Committee had decided, a Sterilization Bill[2] was drafted in 1932 (Müller 1985, 127f).

> For a person who is sick with hereditary mental disease, hereditary feeblemindedness, hereditary epilepsy, or who possesses its hereditary character, an operation of sterilization may be performed, if he himself consents to it and a severe physical or mental hereditary disease can be predicted with a high probability (Section 1).

Sterilization was allowed after the approval of a committee, consisting of two physicians with German medical qualification and a judge of the guardian court. One of the physicians was required to be an expert in human genetics (Section 4). A petition for sterilization could be presented to the committee by the person himself, by his legal representative, a physician, or the director of a hospital or institution (Section 2).

Many German physicians reacted affirmatively towards this bill. The Protestant Inner Mission agreed on the condition that sterilization would be applied only to a person with no relatives, while the Catholic Church and its Caritas (social welfare organization) were firmly opposed to the bill on the basis of Pius XI's papal encyclical *Casti connubii*[3] of December 31, 1930, which absolutely denounced all negative eugenics, including sterilization and abortion[4] (Kawashima, 1993/1997, 294-297; Kawashima, 2004). This bill vanished, however, in the confusion of Prussian coup d'état and the Nazi's grasp of political power on January 30, 1933 (See Müller, 101, 103, 105).

1. 世界恐慌　　2. プロイセン断種法案
3. 教皇ピウス 11 世の回勅「カスティ・コンヌビイ」　　4. 人工妊娠中絶

5. Eugenic Racism of Adolf Hitler

It is well-known that Adolf Hitler[1] and his comrades devoted themselves to ultra racism,[2] that is, Nordic idolization and the principle of the struggle for existence. For Hitler, only the German "*Volk*" (folk),[3] which consisted of the Nordic race,[4] was qualified to reign over the world. For this reason, it was considered necessary to purify the German nation, that is, to exterminate the "Jewish bacilli," to exclude inferior elements and unworthy persons from the German *Volk*, and to promote the human betterment of the German race. He wrote in his book *Mein Kampf*[5] [My Struggle]:

> [The folkish State] has to take care that only the healthy beget children; that there is only one disgrace: to be sick and bring children into the world despite one's own deficiencies; but one highest honor: to renounce this.... Thereby the State has to appear as the guardian of a thousand year's future.... It has to put the most modern medical means at the service of this knowledge. It has to declare unfit for propagation everybody who is visibly ill and has inherited disease and it has to carry this out in practice. (Hitler 1925/1926, 446f; 1941, 608).

6. Nazi Sterilization Law

In 1933, the first year of the Nazi Regime, the Expert Committee of Population and Race drafted a sterilization law. Its members were Hans F. K. Guenther[6] (professor of socio-anthropology), Alfred Ploetz (eugenicist), Gerhard Wagner[7] (chairman of Nazi Doctor Association), Heinrich Himmler[8] (national head of the Gestapo and the SS), Ernst Rüdin (psychiatrist), Fritz Lenz[9] (professor of race hygiene), Richard-Walther Darré[10] (Reich leader for farmers) and Fritz Thyssen[11] (industrialist) (ARGB 1933, 27, 419f).

On July 14, 1933, Hitler's cabinet enacted the *Gesetz zur Verhütung erbkranken Nachwuchses*[12] [Law for the Prevention of Hereditarily Diseased Offspring (Nazi Sterilization Law)] and put it into force on January 1, 1934. The purposes of this legislation, according to Home Minister Wilhelm Frick's[13] comments in a cabinet document, were the prevention of propagation of less worthy persons, the purification of the body of the folk (eugenic racism), the reduction of social and medical expenditures, and the need for neighborly love (ARGB 1933, 27, 412-419). Regulations in Section 1 of this law are as follows:

(1) Anyone with hereditary disease[14] may be rendered sterile by surgical means,

---

1. アドルフ・ヒトラー 2. 人種主義 3. 民族 4. 北方人種 5. 『わが闘争』
6. ハンス・F・K・ギュンター 7. ゲルハルト・ヴァグナー 8. ハインリヒ・ヒムラー
9. フリッツ・レンツ 10. リヒァルト=ヴァルター・ダレ 11. フリッツ・ティッセン
12. 遺伝病子孫予防法（ナチス断種法） 13. ヴィルヘルム・フリック 14. 遺伝病

when, according to medical experience, it is highly probable that the offspring of such a person will suffer from severe inherited mental or bodily disorders.

(2) The law applies to all who suffer from any of the following diseases: 1. Congenital feeblemindedness[1] 2. Schizophrenia[2] (dementia praecox) 3. Manic-depressive insanity[3] 4. Inherited epilepsy[4] 5. Huntington's chorea[5] 6. Hereditary blindness,[6] 7. Hereditary deafness[7] 8. Severe hereditary malformation.[8]

(3) In addition, anyone with severe alcoholism[9] may be sterilized.

According to Section 3, sterilization could also be recommended by a medical officer or the institution director for inmates of a hospital, sanatorium, nursing home or prison. That meant compulsory sterilization. The Eugenic Court[10] of the district had legal jurisdiction in such cases. The court consisted of a Magistrate as chairman, an official physician, and another physician licensed to practice in Germany, who was especially conversant with the principles of eugenics (Section 6) (*Reichsgesetzblatt*, Teil 1, 1933, Nr.86, 529-531; Gütt/Rüdin/Ruttke 1934, 56-59).

In the Nazi period until 1945, some 300,000 to 400,000 persons were sterilized under this law, that is, approximately 0.5% of the German population or one in 200 persons. After 1939, the number of sterilized persons decreased greatly because the secret Euthanasia Action began to exterminate the disabled and mental patients, and an estimated 200,000 persons were killed by gas and other means. Many countries had and have sterilization laws, but the number of victims of this law in Nazi Germany far outnumbers that of any other country.*3

In postwar Germany, financial aid was provided to survivors of compulsory sterilization. In 1980, an amount of 5,000 DM was paid as compensation,[11] and since 1990 a pension of 1,000 DM has been delivered monthly. An allowance of 5,000 DM was also paid to the families of Euthanasia Action victims (Satō 1993, 422-424).*4

7. National Eugenic Law in Japan

Eugenics was also introduced in Japan, especially from England and America from the end of the 19th century, and spread among intellectuals. They promoted eugenic thought, and also proposed eugenic legislation, including sterilization. The eugenic legislative movement intensified after 1933 after learning of the Nazi Sterilization Law, because Japan was rapidly approaching Germany as a similar totalitarian state. This Law was translated and introduced soon afterwards in Japan.*5

Fujimoto Sunao,[12] professor of law, wrote in his 1941 book *Danshu hō*[13]

1. 先天性精神薄弱　2. 精神分裂病（統合失調症）　3. そううつ病
4. 遺伝性てんかん　5. ハンチントン病　6. 遺伝性盲　7. 遺伝性聾
8. 重度の遺伝性奇形　9. 重度のアルコール中毒（依存症）
10. 優生裁判所（遺伝健康裁判所）　11. 補償　12. 藤本直　13. 『断種法』

[Sterilization Law]:

Advocating the necessity of legislating sterilization is not a new idea. It came to our attention several years ago that Germany had put a sterilization law in force on January 1, 1934 and sterilized nearly sixty thousand persons in a year, and that the results were very good. This became a great impetus for us Japanese. In 1936 Japan and Germany entered into the Anti-Comintern Pact[1] and our friendship was greatly strengthened. The fact that Germany is making strong efforts to implement sterilization spurred on the sterilization movement in our country (Fujimoto 1941, 326 and cf. 356).

In 1940 Japan and Germany formed an Axis alliance with fascist Italy under the Tripartite Pact,[2] which was hostile to England and America.

The National Eugenic Law[3] was enacted on May 1, 1940 and put in force on July 1, 1941. The aim of this law was written in Section 1:

This law has the aim of national betterment by preventing the increase of persons with bad hereditary characteristics and by intending to increase the persons with healthy characteristics (Koseisho Yobokyoku, 1941a, 1).

The measure to prevent the reproduction of the hereditarily diseased was sterilization, which was called "eugenic operation"[4] in this law. The substance of this law was, therefore, a sort of sterilization law which was similar to the German law. According to the explanation of Minister of Health and Welfare Yoshida Shigeru,[5,*6] the reason for this legislation was a negative eugenic intention (See Fujimoto 1941, p.262f). Japan and Germany shared the same awareness of crisis that an increase in hereditary patients causes the degeneration of the race and the fall of the state. The racial eugenic thought of human betterment and development of the state was similar in Japan and Germany.

"The Commentary of the National Eugenic Law" published in 1941 by the Ministry of Health and Welfare[6] presented the German situation.

With the establishment of the Nazi Regime, the belief of German folk state has become the national principle; race hygiene has become the basis of all policies; the plentiful reproduction of healthy and fit Germans is the first purpose. ... Hitler appeared and propagated to the utmost the purity and development of the folk. Now, gradually, the effects are beginning to appear (Koseisho Yobokyoku 1941b,

1. 日独防共協定　2. 日独伊三国同盟　3. 国民優生法　4. 優生手術　5. 吉田茂
6. 厚生省

8f).

In this sentence an expectation is shown that in Japan the same effect could be achieved, if a eugenic policy like that of the Nazis were to be adopted.

The National Eugenic Law called sterilization a "eugenic operation" (Section 2). Section 3 regulated the targeted diseases of sterilization: 1. Hereditary mental disease, 2. Hereditary feeblemindedness, 3. Severely bad abnormal hereditary characteristics, 4. severely bad inherited diseases, 5. Severe hereditary deformity (Koseisho Yobokyoku 1941a, 1; 1941b, 1 and 26).

The list of diseases in the National Eugenic Law is general and summary, while the regulation of the Nazi Sterilization Law is concrete and individual. But it is evident that the Japanese includes all diseases covered in the German law, although the latter regulates alcoholics which the former excludes.

Not only the person concerned but also his parents, husband or wife, guardian, or the director of a mental hospital or health center could make the application for sterilization (Section 4 and 5). An application for a eugenic operation could be accepted even without necessary consent if considered to be indispensable (Section 6), which means compulsory sterilization.

The power to rule on sterilization after application belonged to the official chief of the concerned district. He had to elicit the opinion of the eugenic judging committee before making his decision (Section 8). The applicant could raise an objection to the decision with the Minister of Health and Welfare, who had to seek the opinion of the Central Eugenic Judging Committee (Section 10). The decision procedure of sterilization in Japan was different from that in Germany and easier than in Germany (Koseisho Yobokyoku 1941a, 2-5 ; 1941b, 2f. and 33-39).

The Japanese Law has a clause for compulsory sterilization in the Section 6 as stated above. But, in practice, this clause was suspended, and only voluntary sterilization was performed under this law. The National Eugenic Law in Japan did not introduce artificial abortion and castration[1] of sexual offenders which were adopted in the revision of the Nazi Sterilization Law on May 26, 1935 (Gütt/Rüdin/Ruttke, 1936, 80). The Criminal Law of Japan prohibited abortion[2] in the sections 212-216. Under the National Eugenic Law only 538 persons were sterilized between 1941 and 1948 (Yūseishujutsu ni taisuru shazai wo motomerukai 2003, 141). Japan needed many soldiers and children in the Asian Pacific War[3], especially until 1945. One of the popular slogans at that time was: "Be fruitful and multiply!"[4] (See Asahi Shimbun 2010, 159-168).

In 1945, Germany and then Japan accepted an unconditional surrender, and the

1. 去勢   2. 堕胎罪   3. アジア・太平洋戦争   4. 「産めよ殖やせよ」

regime of fascism fell. In postwar Germany, eugenic thought and policy has been connected with Nazism, even though the Sterilization Law was not immediately abolished, but only suspended. On the contrary in postwar Japan, eugenic policy was strengthened: its legal appearance was the Eugenic Protection Law[1] of 1948 (See Yonemoto et al. 2004, 186-190). One can say, therefore, that the influence of Nazi Germany's Sterilization Law upon Japan was stronger after the war than during the war.

8. In Postwar Japan

In the second half of 19th century and into the 20th century, eugenic thought and policy spread and under this background the sterilization laws were enacted in western countries. This tendency, especially the Nazi Sterilization Law of 1933 had a decisive influence on Japanese legislation. The National Eugenic Law of 1940 introduced only voluntary sterilization, and the number of sterilized persons was limited because abundant reproduction and a large population was regarded as necessary for victory in war.

After World War II,[2] eugenic policy in Japan was strengthened in order to stop the drastic increase in population. For this purpose, the Eugenic Protection Law, which aimed at "preventing the birth of bad offspring," was enacted in 1948 instead of the National Eugenic Law (Section 1).

This Law introduced compulsory sterilization and abortion for persons with mental disease (schizophrenia, manic-depression, epilepsy, Huntington's chorea), feeblemindedness, deformity, leprosy, sexual offense, habitual criminality, and twenty other diseases (*Roppō Zensho*, 1995, 3158-3160).

Under this Law some 16,500 persons were sterilized without their consent from 1948 to 1996. This law and also the Leprosy Prevention Law[3] were abolished at long last in 1996. In 1997 the representatives of 17 groups of the disabled and women brought a demand for apology and compensation for compulsory sterilization under the Eugenic Protection Law to the Ministry of Health and Welfare. The Ministry refused this demand, because everything was carried out according to the law (*Asahi Shimbun*, Sept. 17, 1997; Cf. *Yūseishujutsu ni taisuru shazai wo motomerukai* 2003, 216-229). The Japanese State apologized only to the ex-patients of Hansen's disease[4] and compensated them for the long-time infringement of their human rights, because they had won a suit against the state in 2001 (See Kawashima, 2006, p. 23f). The new *Botai Hogohō* [Maternal Protection Law][5] of 1996, which is a drastic revision of the former Eugenic Protection Law, eliminated two-thirds of all clauses, including eugenic words and

1. 優生保護法　2. 第二次世界大戦　3. らい予防法　4. ハンセン病
5. 母体保護法

phrases, for example, "compulsory sterilization" and "forced abortion" (*Roppō Zensho*, 1999, 3494; see Kawashima, 2006, 20ff).

With the enactment of the Maternal Protection Law, the legal remnants of the Nazi Sterilization Law disappeared at long last, but the deep wounds and traumas of sufferers will remain until an official apology and compensation by the state is realized.

Notes

*1 The catechism of the Catholic Church (second edition) reads: "Excessive intervention by the state can threaten personal freedom and initiative. The teaching of the Church has elaborated the principle of *subsidiarity* according to which 'a community of a higher order should not interfere in the internal life of a community of a lower order, depriving the latter of its functions, but rather should support it in case of need and help to co-ordinate its activity with the activities of the rest of society, always with a view of the common good.'" (Part 3, Section 1, Chapter 2, Article 1, 1883).
*2 See Engs 2005; Kawashima 1994/1997 and 2004; Nowak 1984; Thomann 1985; Weindling 2010.
*3 See Bock, 1986; Kawashima, 1993/1994; Klee, 1983; Nowak, 1984.
*4 The 1980 German mark-Japanese yen exchange rate was 1DM = ¥125.
*5 See, for example, my other essay in this book: Chapter 3 "Eugenic Thought of Abe Isoo," esp. 50ff ; For a translation of Nazi Sterilization Law, see *Yūsei Danshuhō to wa nanika*, 1938, 21-42.
*6 He is a different individual from postwar Prime Minister Yoshida Shigeru.

References

Asahi Shimbun ［朝日新聞 Fukuoka-ed.］. Sept. 17, 1997. "Honnin no dōi nashi no funin shujutsu" ［本人の同意なしの不妊手術 Sterilization with consent］.
Asahi Shimbun. 2010. *Shimbun to "Showa"* (新聞と「昭和」Newspapers and "Showa") 2010. Tokyo: Asahi Shimbun Shuppan.
Binding, Karl; Hoche, Alfred. 1920. *Die Freigabe der Vernichtung lebensunwerten Lebens: Ihr Mass und ihre Form*. Leipzig: Felix Meiner.
Bock, Gisela. 1986. *Zwangssterilisation im Nationalsozialismus. Studien zur Rassenpolitik und Frauenpolitik* ［Compulsory sterilization in Naziism: Studies in race politics and women's politics］. Opladen: Westdeutscher.
Engs, Ruth Clifford. 2005. *The Eugenics Movement: An Encyclopedia*. Westport: Greenwood Press.
Fujimoto Sunao ［藤本直］. 1941. *Danshuhō* ［断種法 Sterilization Law］. Tokyo: Iwanami

Shoten.

Gütt, Arthur/ Rüdin, Ernst/ Ruttke, Falk ed. 1934 and 1936. *Gesetz zur Verhütung erbkranken Nachwuchses* ［Law for the Prevention of Hereditarily Diseased Offspring］. München: Lehmann.

Hitler, Adolf. 1935. *Mein Kampf* ［My Struggle］, 158-159. Aufl. München: Frz. Eher Nachf. (English translation 1941. New York: Reynal & Hitchcock 〈http://www.archive.org/details/meinkampf035176mbp〉.

Hoffmann, Géza von. 1913. *Die Rassenhygiene in den Vereinigten Staaten von Nordamerika* ［Race hygiene in the United States of North America］. München: Lehmann.

Juliusburger, Otto. 1912. "Zur Frage der Kastration und Sterilisation von Verbrechern und Geisteskranken" ［On the question of castration and sterilization of criminals and the mentally ill］ in *Deutsche Medizinische Monatsschrift* 9 (Sonderdruck), 6f.

Kawashima Sachio ［河島幸夫］. 1993/1997 *Sensō, Nachizumu, Kyōkai* ［戦争・ナチズム・教会 War, Nazism, the Church］. Tokyo: Shinkyō Shuppansha.

──── 2004. "Nachisu Yūseiseisaku to kirisuto kyōkai" ［ナチス優生政策とキリスト教会 Nazi Eugenic Policy and Christian Churches］ in *Seimei no rinri* ［生命の倫理］, Yamazaki Kiyoko ［山崎喜代子編］ ed., 235-270. Fukuoka: Kyushu Daigaku Shuppankai.

────. 2006. "Botai hogohō no Nachisuteki keifu?" ［母体保護法のナチス的系譜？ Nazi Geneology of Maternal Protection Law?］ T*he Seinan Law Review* ［西南学院大学法学論集］ 38:3＋4, 1-33.

────. 2013. "Nachisu yūseiseisaku to Nihon eno eikyō" ［ナチス優生政策と日本への影響 Nazi Eugenic Policy and its Influence on Japan］ in *Seimei no Rinri 3* ［生命の倫理 3 Ethics of Life 3］, Yamazaki Kiyoko ［山崎喜代子］, ed., 193-222. Fukuoka: Kyushu Daigaku Shuppankai.

Klee, Ernst. 1983. "*Euthanasie*" *im NS-Staat: Die* "*Vernichtung lebensunwerten Lebens*" ［Euthanasia in the Nazi state: the extermination of those unworthy of life］. Frankfurt/M.: S. Fischer.

Kōseishō Yobōkyoku ［厚生省予防局］. 1941a. *Kokumin Yūseihō ni kansuru hōki oyobi jōki* ［国民優生法に関する法規及条規 Regulations and clauses about National Eugenic Law］ Tokyo: Kōseishō Yobōkyoku ［Dept of Prevention in the Ministry for Health and Welfare］.

────. 1941b. *Kokumin Yūseihō Shakugi* ［国民優生法釈義 Commentary of National Eugenic Law］. Tokyo: Koseisho Yobokyoku.

Kühl, Stefan. 1994. *The Nazi Connection: eugenics, American racism, and German national socialism.* New York: Oxford Univ. Press.

Lex Zwickau ［Law of Zwickau］. 1925. *Bundesarchiv Koblenz* R86/2374. (For English translation see 〈http://germanhistorydocs.ghi-dc.org/pdf/eng/EDU_ZWICKAU_ENG.pdf〉).

Minzoku Eisei Kenkyūkai, ed. ［民族衛生研究会］. 1938. *Yūsei Danshuhō to wa nanika* ［優生

断種法トハ何カ What is the eugenic sterilization law?]. Tokyo: Koseisho Yobokyoku Yuseika.

Müller, Johannes. 1985. *Sterilisation und Gesetzgebung bis 1933* [Sterilization and legislation until 1933]. Husum: Matthiessen. (Anhang: Entwurf des Preussischen Landesgesunheitsamtes für ein Sterilisierungsgesetz vom Juli 1932 [Appendix: Draft of the Prussian state health department for a sterilization law of July 1932]).

Norgren, Tiana. 2001. *Abortion before Birth Control: the Politics in Postwar Japan*. Princeton: Oxford University Press.

Nowak, Kurt. 1984. *'Euthanasie' und Sterilisierung im 'Dritten Reich': Die Konfrontation der evangelischen und katholischen Kirche mit dem 'Gesetz zur Verhütung erbkranken Nachwuchses' und der 'Euthanasie'-Aktion* ["Euthanasia" and sterilization in the "Third Reich": the confrontation of the Protestant and Catholic Churches with the "Law for the Prevention of Hereditarily Diseased Offspring"]. Göttingen: Vandenhoeck & Ruprecht.

Ploetz, Alfred, ed. 1904-1944. *Archiv für Rassen- und Gesellschafts-Biologie einschliesslich Rassen- und Gesellschafts-Hygiene (ARGB)* [Archive for Racial and Social Biology].

Roppō Zensho. [六法全書 A Compendium of laws]. 1995 and 1999. Tokyo: Yuhikaku.

Satō Takeo [佐藤健生]. 1993. "Doitsu no Sengohoshō Rippō to sono jikkō ni tsuite" [ドイツの戦後補償立法とその実行について Compensation and fulfillment in Legislation of Postwar Germany] in *Dorei ika: Doitsu kigyō no sengosekinin* [奴隷以下―ドイツ企業の戦後責任 Less than Slaves: Postwar responsibility of German Enterprises], 424-470. (Original title by Benjamin Frenz 1979). Tokyo: Gaifusha..

Thomann, Klaus-Dieter. 1985. "Auf dem Weg in den Faschismus" [On the way to fascism] in *Medizin, Faschismus und Widerstand* [Medicine, facism and resistance], 15-185. Barbara Bromberger, et al., ed. Köln: Pahl-Rugenstein.

Weindling, Paul. 2010. "German eugenics and the wider world: Beyond the racial state" in Alison Bashford and Philippa Levine, ed. *The Oxford Handbook of the History of Eugenics*, 315-331. Oxford : Oxford University Press.

Wollasch, Hans-Joseph. 1978. *Beiträge zur Geschichte der deutschen Caritas in der Zeit der Weltkriege* [Contributions to the history of the German Caritas in the time of the World Wars]. Freiburg i. Br.: Deutscher Caritasverband.

Yonemoto Shōhei/Matsubara Yōko/Nudeshima Jirō/Ichinokawa Yasutaka [米本昌平/松原洋子/ 橳島次郎/市野川容孝]. 2004. *Yūseigaku to Ningen Shakai* [優生学と人間社会 Eugenics and Human Sociedty]. Tokyo: Kōdansha Gendaishinsho.

Yūsei shujutsu ni taisuru shazai wo motomeru kai, ed. [優生手術に対する謝罪を求める会]. 2003. *Yūseihogohō ga okashita tsumi* [優生保護法が犯した罪 Crimes committed by the Eugenic Protection Law]. Tokyo: Gendaishokan.

Part III

Implementation of Eugenics in Japan

Chapter 7

Eugenics: Its Spread and Decline

Chūman Mitsuko

The historical study of eugenics and eugenic thought in the formative process of contemporary Japan is very important when considering the most up to date bioethical problems. The history of eugenics and eugenic thought in Japan before World War II can be divided into three periods. 1) Early Meiji Period[1] (1880s): European and American ideas were imported and discussion of the racial improvement of Japanese through intermarriage with other races began. 2) Mid-Meiji Period[2] (1890s): As eugenics and eugenic thought was brought in from Europe and America, its popularity gradually spread among Japanese as a leading-edge academic discipline. 3) Late Taishō Period[3] (1910s): A eugenics research system was developed, and the enlightenment movement became widespread. The national management of "human resources"[4] was connected to eugenics under the total war and general mobilization system, resulting in the enactment of the National Eugenic Law.[5]

Postwar history can also be summarized in three periods. 1) Period from 1948: The Eugenic Protection Law[6] was enacted, and abortion of pregnancy was legalized. Postwar governmental eugenic policies were enacted practically on legal grounds. 2) Period from 1970: With the rapid development of life sciences and reproductive medicine, the urgent need to establish bioethics began to be recognized. From the viewpoint of defending the human rights and reproduction rights of persons with disabilities, traditional eugenic thought and practices became relativized or considered taboo. 3) Period from 2003: After the success of decoding the human genome, a time of new genetics and new eugenics began. Eugenic selection began spreading among people based on the development of techniques for prenatal genetic diagnosis.

This chapter will analyze the Meiji, Taishō, and Shōwa periods before World War II in order to clarify details of the birth of eugenics and eugenic though in contemporary Japan.

---

1. 明治初期　2. 明治中期　3. 大正後期　4. 「人的資源」の国家管理
5. 国民優生法　6. 優生保護法

1. The Emergence of Eugenics in the Development of Modern Japanese Hygiene

a) Hygiene and eugenics—the Road to strengthening the nation

The influence of the theory of social evolution on the theory of modern hygiene[1] becomes conspicuous mainly in writings from around the 1890s. The principle of the survival of the fittest (the strong win, the weak lose[2]) became the principle for evaluating the state of the nation's health as a whole. One example is Gotō Shinpei's *Kokka eisei genron*[3] [Principles of National Hygiene] from 1889, in which he maintained that Darwinian evolution could function as the principle of national hygiene. Guarding health and preserving life evolved as the common responsibility of both the nation and its individual citizens.

Hygiene in this early period was considered to be a vital pillar in ensuring a healthy work force, in promoting industry from the standpoint of guaranteeing a viable military force, and in enriching the nation and strengthening the army. To achieve this, provincial administrative organization of the police force was necessary. People were afraid of the policemen, who, for the purpose of disinfection and quarantine,[4] raided their homes and sent family members off to the quarantine hospitals, without allowing protest. The quarantine hospitals were hospitals in name only. Medical care was seldom administered, and very few survived to return to their homes.

In the late Meiji period, which showed a decrease in acute infectious diseases, policies were added which valued the maintenance of societal peace and order, as well as Japan's international reputation. This can be seen in venereal disease examinations under the enactment of the *Shōgi torishimari kisoku*[5] [Regulation for the Control of Prostitutes], the establishment of the Mental Patients' Custody Act,[6] the promulgation of food sanitation laws,[7] and the passage of the tuberculosis prevention ordinance[8] and the leprosy prevention law.[9] In regards to labor hygiene, Gotō Shinpei founded and chaired the occupational hygiene investigation group,[10] published "Shokukō jijyō"[11] [Workers' Conditions], and got the Factory Act passed. A health insurance law was approved as a social administrative policy to deal with the economic depression of World War I, strikes, and tenant disputes. In a manner of speaking, from the stage of pursuing only the treatment of acute infectious diseases emerged a stage of improving national nutritional, health, and sanitation conditions and preventing the onset of disease. However, at the same time, there was a "national hygiene"[12] policy based on eugenic thought which needed "human resources," that is to say, healthy bodies of people who possessed the mental and technical abilities required by the nation.

The hygiene policy, which began as communicable disease control infrastructure,[13]

1. 衛生思想成立過程   2. 優勝劣敗   3. 後藤新平『国家衛生原理』   4. 消毒・隔離
5. 娼妓取締規則   6. 精神病者監護法   7. 食品衛生   8. 肺結核予防令
9. 癩予防法   10. 職業衛生調査会   11. 職工事情   12. 民族衛生   13. 防疫体制

was mainly administered by the urban and rural prefectural police departments, who were responsible for police crackdowns.[1] But as the Shōwa era began, the focus shifted to improving the national physical condition. In the process of establishing a modern state, it can be said that the administrative police pressed for adaptation and assimilation to the national order and controlled people's lives[2] by preventing deviation from or rebellion against the national order. Administration of hygiene also came into existence, working closely with such administrative police methods. The inherent basic principle of eugenic thought emphasized this aspect of national policy. It can be said that the fundamental basis of Western hygiene studies—such as citizen autonomy and the emphasis on human nature in "public hygiene"—was weakened.

b) International expositions and japonism—People on display

An International Exposition, which proposed to collect human wisdom and show the peak of civilization, was held for the first time in London in 1861. Starting from that year, the second half of the nineteenth century plunged into an "Era of International Expositions."[3] The Tokugawa shogunate, the Satsuma clan, and the Saga clan participated in the 1867 Paris International Exposition, but Japan's first participation as a nation was in the 1873 Austrian International Exposition in Vienna. From that time on, Japan began to hungrily acquire Western culture.

Beginning with the 1889 Paris Exposition, "human exhibits"[4]—the exhibition of the natives of colonies and settlements—were held. These exhibits reflected the principle of white dominance and justified colonization. They also became a means of creating the image of a wealthy empire. Japan also held many exhibits which encouraged Western Japonism. On the other hand, Japan, legitimatized its own superiority and colonization with such exhibits as the Taiwan Pavilion, the Korean Museum, and exhibits of Ainu settlements.[5,*1] At that time it was widely held that the Ainu ethnic group was a "perishing race." Fujino points out that the Nazis, in order to maintain the myth of "Aryan race" superiority, put eugenic policies in place which would eliminate intermarriage with other ethnic groups, especially the Jews. In contrast, Japan, based on the logic of enhancing their characteristics, promoted intermarriage with the Ainu and others in its colonies and occupied areas (Fujino 1998, 258-259). Hirota also maintains that anthropology created a discriminatory viewpoint[6] that can be clearly seen in the Osaka Domestic Industrial Exhibition's anthropology exhibit.[*2] According to the logic of modern civilization, the greater part of the discriminatory viewpoint of our modern eyes came into existence during the hundred years and some decades since the Meiji period. However, the warning from this event seems to be that the source of discrimination lies rather in the social structure of our own lives (Hirota 1998, 101-103).

1. 警察的取締 2. 民衆生活を統制 3. 万国博覧会の時代 4. 人間の展示
5. アイヌ民族 6. 差別の視線

Sakanishi also points out that in the process of clarifying the psychological and historical background which gave shape to modern Japan's racial stereotype[1] and prejudice, "the surging waves of Western culture and civilization" and sudden contact with "different races"[2] gave birth to a uniform view and attitude toward race in Japan, resulting in a stereotype of white, black, and yellow peoples[3] (Sakanishi 2005, iv). In other words, the racial and ethnic consciousness of Japanese at that time was subservient and accommodating toward Western Caucasians, as opposed to arrogant, scornful, and condescending toward Asians. It is thinkable that such attitudes have been carried over even to this day.

The opening of the era of expositions meant the start of the information age in which the history of man could first be experienced. Exhibitions were the place where Japan sought to assimilate not only information about industrialization,[4] but also information about all of Western civilization.[5] The assimilation of much of that information, as a matter of course, was carried over into multifaceted domestic reform.

c) Hygiene exhibit and the Red Cross Archive—Superior heredity and marriage

Ono Yoshirō notes that the Greater Japan Private Hygiene Association[6] played a large role in the popularization of equipment for the hygiene system, that popular lectures served as the tip end of an antenna for the hygiene system, and that hygiene exhibitions[7] functioned as visual media[8] (Ono 1997, 134).

In fact, Kobashi Ichita made the following observations in print:

> There are various means of promoting hygienic thought among the people. But I would say, first of all, the most concrete and most appropriate are the "Hygiene Exhibitions" that were held throughout the country starting last year or the publication of "Pictures of Hygienic Activities"[9] from the "Hygiene lectures"[10] for the common people to read. These are the methods that absolutely have to be employed. ... "The development of public health administration" and "the spread of hygienic ideas,"[11] must develop along with civic responsibility, and must be sunk deeply into the minds of municipal residents... (Kobashi 1912, 477-481).

Tanaka Satoshi points out that the large-scale, enlightenment hygiene exhibitions were part of expositions in which eight entities participated—the Greater Japan Private Hygiene Association, the Red Cross Museum,[12] the Home Ministry, the Education Ministry, local governments, private companies such as newspapers, and the police. From the content of the exhibits and the history of hygienic exhibitions, he tries to investigate how the ideas of the "body"[13] were changed and, in that change, how people

---

1. 人種ステレオタイプ　　2. 異人種　　3. 白人・黒人・黄色人　　4. 産業化
5. 西洋文明　　6. 大日本私立衛生学会　　7. 衛生展覧会　　8. 視覚メディア
9. 衛生活動写真　　10. 衛生講話会　　11. 衛生思想の普及　　12. 赤十字博物館
13. 身体

came under the control of the authorities (Tanaka 1994, 29-30).

The Greater Japan Private Hygiene Association, at time of its fifth annual meeting held the first "Hygiene Specimen Exhibition"[1] at Tokyo's Tsukiji Hongan-ji Temple. It was so well attended that the three day event was extended another day. After that for the next ten years, an exhibition was held several times in conjunction with the annual meeting.

In April 1894, the Greater Japan Private Hygiene Association held its 12th Annual Meeting in Kyoto.

In conjunction with this, the "Hygiene Specimen Exhibition" was held for five days from April 22 to 26 at the Teramachi-Dōri special teacher-training school. Included were samples of human body elements (Tokyo Hygiene Laboratory), chemical analysis results table related to hygiene (Osaka Private Hygiene Society), a vaccination sword (Greater Japan Private Hygiene Association Cowpox Vaccination Center) (*DaiNippon shiritsu eiseikai* 132 (May 26, 1894), 469-574).

In 1926, an "archive"[2] was established on the grounds of the Japan Red Cross Headquarters in Tokyo's Shibadaimon (Japan Red Cross Society 1995, 231).*[3] In 1932, it became the "Red Cross Museum"[3] and put much effort into hygiene enlightenment activities until its closing in 1963, due to aging facilities. At its 50th anniversary celebration, the Japan Red Cross Society established a "museum to gain the respect of the world." It was introduced as having a complete collection of common useful hygiene goods—"from food, shelter, and clothing, in general, to specific medical goods related to pregnancy, childbirth and child raising, eugenics or race hygiene, and nursing care for illness.

At the "Ethnic Hygiene Exhibition"[4] (1928) two years after the opening of the museum, the opening statement of purpose read:

> ... accompanying the advances of recent industrial development society, the so-called "civilized diseases"[5] of tuberculosis, venereal disease, feeblemindedness, and alcohol addiction are becoming stronger with a violent force in our country, and the number of deaths particularly among infants, toddlers, and women of childbearing age[6] shows a high rate rarely seen in other countries. In addition, because the birth of mentally deficient and disabled persons with bad genes is flourishing, compared with that of superior classes of ability, inferior unfit genes are on the increase. That the condition of the talent of our nation is in this way gradually decreasing is a matter of unending concern for the future of our state (Japan Red Cross 1928).

1. 衛生参考品展覧会　2. 参考館　3. 赤十字博物館　4. 民族衛生展覧会
5. 文明病　6. 乳幼児出産期婦人の死亡数

According to the archive bulletin, four of the seven corners of the exhibit were "National deterioration and population statistics,"[1] "Materials concerning human genetics,"[2] "Materials on sex-linked inheritance,"[3] and "Materials concerning the harms of alcohol and industrial development and national health."[4] These displays put emphasis on providing genetic knowledge. For example, in the fifth corner the "Inheritance of Parents' traits by their offspring," Gregor Mendel and his experiments, along with the results of crossbreeding experiments with chickens, mice, wheat, morning glories, etc., were illustrated. At the sixth corner, "Materials concerning genetics and marriage," there was information about the offspring of General Martin Kallikak, the offspring of Jonathan Edwards, and the genealogy of Japanese authors from the Edo period. The "mentally deficient and lazy" Juke family was also introduced. For this family "for 75 years until 1877 New York state prison and orphanage system had spent a total of $1,250,000. For fifty years their seed had been sown and scattered throughout the United States." Furthermore, at the seventh corner, "Materials concerning national deterioration due to infectious diseases of the people," were exhibits consisting of statistics concerning venereal disease, tuberculosis, as well as Hansen's disease, family trees showing the inheritance of mental illness, and various articles made by patients of mental hospitals.

Next, at the "Marriage Hygiene Exhibition,"[5] held jointly with the Japan Society of Race Hygiene in 1933, the presentation asserted that "even if the achievements of the person in question are somewhat bad, there is no problem if the parents, siblings, aunts and uncles, and grandparents are highly capable. Excellent genetic quality is revealed in the person's offspring." Following a study of bloodlines,[6] engagement should be made after "a mutual exchange of medical health certificates[7] done by a trusted doctor." During the period of the exhibition, Ichikawa Genzō gave a lecture entitled "The Biggest Contradiction in Spouse Selection." In his lecture, Ichikawa gives the following edification:

That most people do not think this way is because we do not educate about eugenics. If the eugenics movement spreads to the point of being a personal morality, or religion, people will not feel other restrictions, but will be able to have eugenic marriages. In any case, it must be said that the spread of eugenics is the prime task at the moment. (Tanaka 1994).

The Ministry of Health and Welfare,[8] strengthening a sense of crisis about population decline, released "The Ten Commandments of Marriage"[9] in September 1939, under the auspices of the Prevention Bureau's National Hygiene Research Group:

1. 民族劣化と人口統計　　2. 人類の遺伝に関する資料　　3. 伴性遺伝に関する資料
4. 酒の害及び産業の発達と民族の健康に関する資料　　5. 結婚衛生展覧会　　6. 血統調査
7. 健康診断書　　8. 厚生省　　9. 結婚十訓

1. Choose a person whom you can trust as a lifelong partner.
2. Choose a person who is both mentally and physically healthy.
3. Choose a person without bad heredity.
4. Avoid marrying blindly.
5. Avoid marriage with close relatives, if at all possible.
6. Avoid marrying late in life.
7. Do not be a slave to superstitions or conventions.
8. Get guidance from parents and elders and act decisively after mature deliberation.
9. Keep the ceremony simple and file the registration document on the same day.
10. Be fruitful and multiply for the sake of the country (Hozumi 1941, 5-186).

The model for the "Ten Commandments of Marriage" was the Nazi "Ten Rules for Spouse Selection." Hereafter, the Ministry of Health and Welfare begin to adopt policies which strongly reflect the Nazi eugenic ideology.

This emphasis can also be seen in the exhibits of Japan National Eugenics Exhibit[1] (1939) which were divided into six corners: "Ethnic Extinction,"[2] "The Light of Japan as the power of a prosperous Asia,"[3] "Crisis of Civilization,"[4] "Ethnic Eugenic Measures,"[5] "Physical Fitness Improvement,"[6] and "The Path of Strengthening the Nation."[7] As the "finale" of the last corner, "The Spirit of Imperial Rule"[8] was heralded, and on the right side of a large picture of a big tree was the Population Problems Research Institute's[9] "Ten Commandments for Strengthening the Nation."[10] Included in these were national policy slogans and exhortations far removed from useful hygiene information: "bear many good children; don't let the children already born die; toughen your body and mind; eradicate tuberculosis and leave behind racial poisons; build healthy and cheerful cities; be careful of the tendency toward vain pleasures; protect the simplicity and fortitude of farming communities; hold firm to Japan's unique family system; abandon individualism for the nation; extol the spirit of Japan throughout the world. In particular, not only were the sickly family lines exposed as inferior stock in the "national eugenic measures," voices were also raised to encourage the increase of superior stock. Around this time, the need for marriage prohibition legislation[11] and sterilization legislation[12] was being emphasized and an explanatory "sterilization and castration"[13] chart was exhibited (Tanaka 1994, 31).

1. 日本民族優生展覧会　2. 民族滅亡　3. 日本の光，興亜の力　4. 文明の危機
5. 民族優生方策　6. 体力向上　7. 民族強化の道　8. 皇道精神
9. 人口問題研究所　10. 民族強化十訓　11. 結婚禁止法　12. 断種法
13. 断種と去勢

2. The Heyday of Eugenics

a) Hygiene proponents' view of marriage

We turn our attention now to the view of marriage of the time. In his *Kon'in heigairon* [Discussion of Marriage Abuse], Nagayo Sensai[1] (Nagayo 1884,1) assumed that marriage not only determines the fortune or misfortune, the honor or disgrace of one's life, but also that sufficient attention should be paid to the fact that the advantages and disadvantages carry over to the future generations of descendants. He explained that sufficient attention should be given to "genetic diseases" like leprosy and epilepsy.[2] He also outlined four prerequisites: age, health, knowledge, conduct or scholarly assets.[3] He evaluated "health" on three levels. The top level for a marriage partner was presented as follows: "A good husband is a man who is handsome in his looks and proportion, muscular, academically active, not rash and frivolous, broad-chested, has a voice that carries well, good vision, a ruddy complexion, and good posture. Just by looking, one can tell that he is a fine man. A good wife is a woman who is beautiful, with a good figure, feminine, healthy, red-cheeked, with a clear voice and a well-developed thorax." Nagayo had a fairly accurate understanding of hereditary disease, but including "handsome looks" or "good figures" in eugenic traits is an interesting point for investigating the later changes in the view of bioethics.

Furthermore, Shimoda Utako[4] defines the purpose of hygiene as not just preventing disease, but also increasing physical strength and longevity. She emphasized that many mentally ill, mentally retarded, blind, and deaf persons were the result of consanguineous marriages[5] and that progeny of early marriages were often frail idiots. The most easily inherited condition was mental disease and nervous disorders, and one needed to pay special attention to the genetic pedigree of felons. In addition, she mentions "accordingly, I think our Japan nation undoubtedly inherited our spirit of loyalty and patriotism from our ancestors" (Shimoda 1906, 1 ,9, 134).

It may well be said that the peak of hygiene theory in this period is summed up in Ogata Masakiyo's[6] book (Ogata 1907, 4, 8, 69, 72, 87, 90, 122, 178, 182, 198). He stressed the importance of selecting a spouse: "the British man Galton published a new theory, the study of good breeding, which "advocates that race improvement can be expected by careful attention to marriage." "Women in civilized countries marry between twenty and forty-five years of age," while "in barbaric countries they are often married by age twelve." The choice for the time of marriage is based on a series of choices, placing importance on "physical characteristics, academic ability, personality, etc." The marriage of "men and women with strong bodies"[7] makes possible the "birth of strong offspring."

---

1. 長與專齋 2. 癩病癲癇などの遺伝病 3. 年齢健康知識品行及び学術資産
4. 下田歌子 5. 血族結婚 6. 緒方正清 7. 強壮なる男女

It is a given that the "marriage of frail men and women"[1] can in the long run only produce frail offspring. In such homes, harmony is also missing or it "causes mental illness or ends in a shortened life for parents and child."

Also, he asserted that it is good that statistics about the "evils of consanguineous marriage"[2] were made public and that "Article 769 of the Civil Code"[3] was passed in our country, forbidding marriages between relatives in the third degree." Concerning the appropriate marriageable age, he said "for a woman twenty-five and for a man 35 or 36" was an ideal age to marry. Further, he came back to the point that compared to the "grand Western women,"[4] the bodies of "undersized Japanese women"[5] have "poor development of sex organs," so that even if they become pregnant, "miscarriage or abortion"[6] takes place making it difficult to bear perfect children. In England and America, artificial pregnancy methods[7] are being proposed, but in countries like France and Germany, this idea is being dismissed. However, the authority of the home is being usurped by infertility. When talking of divorce, a conclusion should be based on the determination of the "cause of infertility"[8] by a thorough examination by a medical doctor and a wide range of measures.

> The real value and significance of women is in their ability become pregnant and bear children. For women, it is necessary for those who have fulfilled their reproductive function to continue to carry out this most valuable function more and more vigorously. In this world, which should progress more and more according to this competition for survival, [we need to] deepen this feeling without disagreement (Ogata 1907, 198).

Thus, preparation to welcome the heyday of eugenics was complete.

b) Race hygiene and the enlightenment movement

Eugenics became popular in Japan as a cutting-edge academic study in the 1910s. Yasuda Tokutarō[9] looked back on this period:

> I also became a fan of the genetics[10] that was in vogue at that time. It was a time that I read books about genetics in English one after another— [Francis] Galton, [Charles] Davenport, Thompson, [Thomas Hunt] Morgan, Johnson, etc. To be sure, genetics and eugenics were most popular in Japan's economic boom during the Great European War. At the root of that popularity was genetics which useful to the so-called upper class and intelligentsia for their class ideology.[11] It was said: we are the superior class because our inherited qualities are superior. On the other

1. 虚弱な男女の結婚　2. 血族結婚の弊害　3. 民法第769条　4. 雄大なる西洋婦人
5. 矮少な日本婦人　6. 流産及び堕胎　7. 人工妊娠法　8. 不妊の原因
9. 安田徳太郎　10. 遺伝学のファン　11. 上流階級と知識階級の階級理論

hand, the inherited qualities of the impoverished class are inferior so their economic inferiority is a hereditary inevitability. (Fujime 1997, 316)

In 1910 (Meiji 43), Unno Yukinori's *Nihon jinshu kaizōron*[1] [On remodeling the Japanese race] urged Japan, which had been victorious in Russo-Japanese war, to make preparations for the future competition for survival with Western countries. Based on Galton's "anti-selection" principle,[2] Unno advocated the necessity of eugenic study and the enforcement of eugenic polices as national policy. He appealed for the pressing need for a remodeling of the Japanese race. The following year in 1911 (Meiji 44), he expressed the following opinion in *Kōkokusaku toshite no jinshu kaizō* [Race remodeling as a national policy][3]:

If only the disabled and the unfit remain behind and all the healthy-bodied are engaged on the battlefield and die, our country will become the Japan Empire of morons, the Japan Empire of the mentally ill, and the Japan Empire of the deaf. Such are the evils of war. In order to care for our sacred oriental Empire, we must avoid a war that would destroy our good traits and reduce our national values (Unno 1911, 13).

On the other hand, Oka Asajirō, in "*Minshu kaizengaku no jissai kachi*"[4] [The real value of ethnic betterment study] (Oka 1911, 153-159), translated eugenics as *minshu kaizengaku* [study of ethnic betterment], instead of *zenshugaku* [study of good breeding], *yūryōshuzokugaku* [study of superior stock], or *jinshukairyōgaku* [study of race betterment]. What he meant by his translation is shown in the following statements:

Twenty some years earlier, even in our country, there was once talk of race betterment, but that race betterment proposed that Japanese intermarry with superior Westerners, and improve the race by adding the blood of Westerners to that of Japanese.... This time the study of ethnic betterment also has the purpose of improving people, but... to put it simply, we should attempt to apply the laws of biology to human society (Oka 1911, 155).

In the 1920s a eugenics research system was developed and the enlightenment began to flourish and reached its peak. Japan Genetics Society president Tanaka Yoshimaro,[5] who left behind achievements in the study of silkworms, wrote such books as *Ningen taishitsu no kaizen ga kyūmu*[6] [The betterment of human physical qualities is urgent] in

---

1. 海野幸徳『日本人種改造論』 2. ゴルトンの逆淘汰 3. 『興国策としての人種改造』
4. 丘浅次郎『民種改善学の実際的価値』 5. 日本遺伝学会会長田中義麿
6. 『人間本質の改善が急務』

1924 (Taishō 12) and in the following year *Yūseigaku kara mita hainichimondai* [Looking at the anti-Japanese problem from eugenics][1], in which he emphasized the urgency and need for the establishment of a eugenics research institute[2] and a research system for the purpose of building the superior essential qualities of the Yamato race.[3]

In the private sector, Gotō Ryūkichi also published *Yūzenikkusu* (later *Yūseigaku* [Eugenics]), the journal of the Japan Eugenics Society in 1924 (Taishō 13).[4] In February of the following year 1925 (Taishō 14), Yamamoto Senji started publication of *Sanji chōsetsu hyōron* [Birth control review], the title of which was changed to *Sei to shakai* [Sex and Society][5] in October. In 1926 (Taishō 15), Ikeda Shigenori inaugurated the Japan Eugenic Exercise/Movement Association's journal *Yūsei Undō* [Eugenics Exercise/ Movement].[6][*4]

In the preface to the first issue of *Yūsei Undō*, Ikeda made the following assertion:

In the future, the Japanese race must stand on the front lines of the world. A race standing on the front lines should be both a mentally and physically healthy, superior one. In order to grow good grass and flowers, it is necessary to have good seeds, a good field, and good maintenance.[7]

His purpose was not just to have good offspring through eugenic marriages.[8] Instead, he had a broad view of eugenics and insisted on improving environmental aspects, establishing social discipline and order, providing a healthy living environment through the development of social medicine, perfecting a unified, rational organization conducive for co-existence and co-prosperity, attempting a thoroughly autonomous spirit and, on top of that, improving education, thus paving the way to make efforts to cultivate the mind and body. He said: "All human beings are equal. ... Everyone wants a long life, and not just a long life, everyone wants to learn to live youthfully forever" (Ikeda 1926, 2). To accomplish such a lifestyle, one should improve one's physical condition and makeup, obtain the elixir for a long life without aging, reform marriage by giving attention to one's choice of a spouse. For the purpose of creating a more livable society, one should fill one's heart with patriotism, reform the Parliament, and expand women's participation in government.

Moreover, "the reason for 'eugenicists' anxiety about marriage' is all due to 'factors of hereditary defects.'"[9]... Let there be no misunderstanding, it because those without hereditary defects do not eliminate those with defects. " This does not apply to tuberculosis, syphilis, and leprosy. Up until now, there was opposition to the birth control movement,[10] but, if surgeries to limit births or contraceptive methods are not

1. 『優生学から見た排日問題』　2. 優生学研究所の設置　3. 大和民族
4. 後藤龍吉『ユーゼニックス』創刊　5. 山本宣治『産児調節評論』
6. 池田林儀『優生運動』　7. よい草花を作るには，よい種子とよい畑とよい手入れ
8. 優生結婚　9. 遺伝的劣弱素因　10. 産児制限

approved, it will be difficult to attain an ideal married life in society. Ikeda asserted birth control is also helpful for this reason (Ikeda 1927, 2).

3. Reconsidering Nagai Hisomu: Enthusiasm for Eugenics and Enlightenment Activities

In order to examine how the thought and practice of eugenics permeated the Japanese public and how it became socially accepted, this section will focus on the discourse and enlightenment activities of Nagai Hisomu,[1] who devoted himself to eugenics and the passage of a sterilization law in Japan.[2] That is, I want to attempt a reinterpretation of Dr. Nagai. He is generally accepted as a leader of the campaign for the sterilization law, but I want to explore why he turned his attentions from physiological research to concentrate on eugenics and sterilization. By focusing on his statements and educational campaign,[3] I hope to "unearth the 'why' buried in historical darkness."

a) Nagai Hisomu: The Ministry of Health and Welfare and media

As the Shōwa period began, Nagai was instrumental in establishing the *Nippon Minzoku Eisei Gakkai* [Japan Society of Race Hygiene] (1930)[4] and was inaugurated as the chairman of the board of directors. Nagai's insistence on using the word "race hygiene" instead of "eugenics" seems to come from the influence of Alfred Ploetz, who introduced Galton's eugenics to Germany using the term "Rassenhygiene."[5] This is evident in his column for the first issue of the society's journal *Minzoku Eisei* [Race Hygiene]: "We take our stand and are determined to advance, having the same concerns as erudite German scholar, Alfred Ploetz, who stands on the front of the fight for race hygiene" (*Minzokueisi* 1 1931). Even though the Japan Society of Race Hygiene selected a physiologist as their chairman of the board, it was an organization committed to a social movement[6] rather than a medically related academic association. Among the members were politicians like Yoshida Shigeru,[7]*[5] and Hatoyama Ichirō,[8] lawyers, people related to the military, journalists, and the founder of the Taishō *Anzen Dai Ichi* [Safety First] campaign Uchida Yoshikichi.[9] As can be seen from the list of members, the principal objective of the organization was enlightenment, or education, rather than research activities.

In 1935 eugenicists centered around Ikeda submitted a sterilization law draft, *Nippon Minzoku Yūsei Hogohō* [Japanese Race Eugenic Protection Act], to the Diet where it was tabled. But Nagai Hisomu and others continued to emphasize the necessity of a sterilization law and submitted a proposal to the Cabinet, eventually resulting in the

---

1. 永井潜   2. 日本の断種法制定運動のリーダー   3. 啓蒙活動
4. 日本民族衛生学会   5. 民族衛生   6. 社会運動を担う組織   7. 吉田茂
8. 鳩山一郎   9. 内田嘉吉

Diet passing the *Minzoku Yūseihō* [National Eugenic Law][1] in 1940. The first article stated: "the purpose of this law is both to defend the nation from an increase in those who have bad genes resulting in hereditary disease and to improve the quality of the nation's citizens by increasing those who have healthy genes." The "enforcement ordinance" and the "enforcement regulations" of the following year outlined the specifics concerning candidates for sterilization surgery. In the same pamphlet was the organizational chart of the Ministry of Health and Welfare Prevention Bureau[2] which illustrated the procedures and the entities involved in the national eugenics process (See figure 1) (Kōseishō Yobōkyoku 1941).

Yomiuri Shimbun's report[3] on the process of the law's passage quoted the purpose of the law (*Yomiuri Shimbun* evening edition Mar. 9, 1940). A previous report of the push to pass sterilization legislation gives insight into the situation at that time. Along with the article was a photograph of Nagai Hisomu with the headlines: "Cut off the source of bad blood"[4] "Ministry of Health finally taking up the 'sterilization law' desired by this generation"[5] (*Yomiuri Shimbun* (Jan. 28, 1938). Though, unlike today, the readership was limited, this newspaper coverage shows that the mass media of the day welcomed the sterilization law as a policy appropriate for the current situation and that Nagai had became a favored child of his generation.

Persons of authority from the military and naval forces, the judiciary, and psychiatric circles gathered for the first Race Hygiene Conference held in the afternoon of April 22, 1938 to begin preparations for promoting the enactment of the law. Absent from those gathered was Nagai Hisomu, who at the time was the dean of the Medical College of Taipei Imperial University. Instead a photograph of Prevention Bureau head Takano[6] appeared in the newspaper with the following copy: "Dr. Takano Rokurō, who has been the leader in bringing the sterilization law to this point, gave the following comments in the "launching address." 'We have finally "rowed" to the point of holding a conference. We must not get in a hurry just because it's a matter of having a problem. I think we need to proceed prudently (*Yomiuri Shimbun* evening edition April 23, 1938).

The main purpose of the National Eugenic Law, a sterilization law, was to defend the nation from an increase of those with bad genes which resulted in hereditary illnesses. It was a law to "take measures to make them unable to reproduce."[7] One of those hereditary diseases was "hereditary mental illness (schizophrenia, manic depression, and epilepsy)."[8] People who were determined to have such an illness were given operations to prevent them from bearing progeny (Katō 1996).

From media reports[9] in newspaper articles, it can be said that Dr. Nagai took a leading role in spreading this way of thinking. Newspaper reports of his lectures dealing

---

1. 国民優生法　2. 厚生省予防局　3. 読売新聞記事　4. 「断て！悪い血の泉」
5. 「時代の欲望『断種法』を厚生省がいよいよ取り上げ」　6. 高野六郎予防局長
7. 「生殖を不能ならしめる手術または処置」　8. 遺伝性精神病（分裂病・躁鬱病・癲癇）
9. メディア報道

國民優生法

國民素質ノ向上

方法: 惡質ナル遺傳性疾患ノ素質ヲ有スル者ノ增加防過（優生手術）

對象

疾患者
- 遺傳性精神病
- 遺傳性精神薄弱
- 強度且惡質ナル遺傳性病的性格
- 強度且惡質ナル遺傳性身體疾患
- 強度ナル遺傳性畸形

其子又ハ孫ノ同一疾患ニ罹ル虞大ナルトキ

但シ優秀ナル素質ヲ併セ有スル場合ハ除ク

擬者: 上記疾患ノ素質ヲ有スルモノ（習慣ニヨリ其ノ同一疾患ニ罹ル虞大ナルトキ）

手續

任意申請	同意申請	強制申請
本人	本人ヲ診療セル精神病院長、保健所長、特ニ指定スル醫師	若シ惡質ナルトキ又ハ配偶者モ惡質ナルトキ等ニテ必要ナル同意ヲ得ルコト能ハサル場合但シ疾患者ノ優生手術ニ限
配偶者父母等ノ同意	本人配偶者父母等ノ同意	
配偶者父母等ノ申請		

判定 → 地方長官 ⇔ 地方優生審查會（審查）
不服申立 → 厚生大臣 ⇔ 中央優生審查會（審査）

手術ノ實施: 特定ノ醫師ニヨリ特定ノ病院ニ於テ **優生手術**

優生手術ヲ受ケタル者ハ結婚ノ相手方ノ請求アリタル場合、手術ヲ受ケタル旨ノ通知義務

方法: 健全ナル素質ヲ有スル者ノ增加（產兒制限ノ排除）

對象: 故サニ生殖不能ナラシメル手術又ハ放射線照射

手段: 禁止

對象: 醫師ノ行フ生殖不能ナラシメル手術若ハ放射線照射又ハ姙娠中絕

手段: 事前ニ他ノ醫師ヨリ其ノ要否ニ關シ意見聽取

手段: 輸出

添付書類
- 健康診斷書
- 遺傳ニ關スル調査書
- 不姙手術ナルコトヲ知ラセル旨醫師ノ証明書

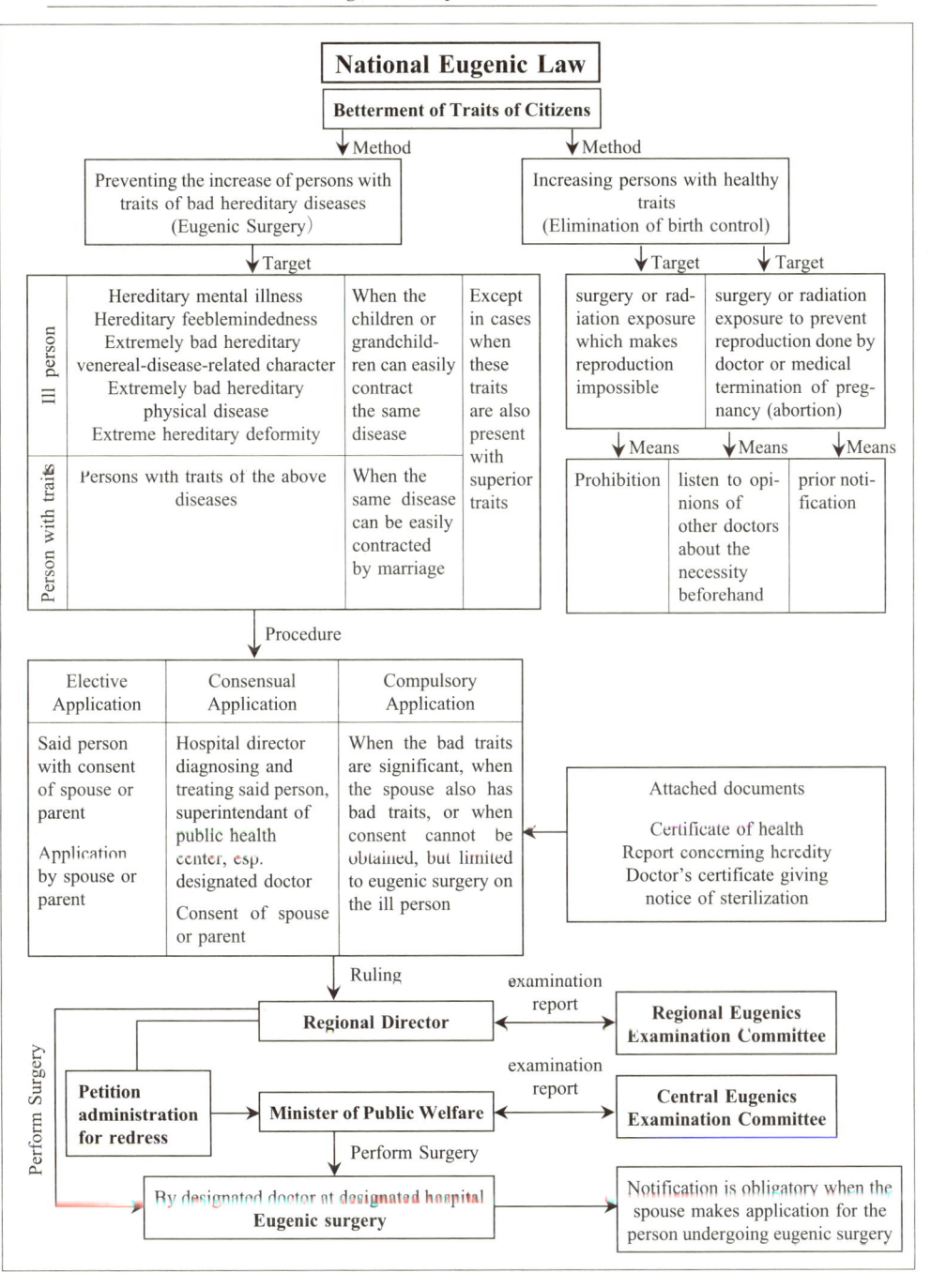

Eugenics: Its Spread and Decline

National Eugenic Law

Betterment of Traits of Citizens

↓ Method: Preventing the increase of persons with traits of bad hereditary diseases (Eugenic Surgery)

↓ Method: Increasing persons with healthy traits (Elimination of birth control)

Target (Preventing)

Ill person	Hereditary mental illness Hereditary feeblemindedness Extremely bad hereditary venereal-disease-related character Extremely bad hereditary physical disease Extreme hereditary deformity	When the children or grandchildren can easily contract the same disease	Except in cases when these traits are also present with superior traits
Person with traits	Persons with traits of the above diseases	When the same disease can be easily contracted by marriage	

Target (Increasing)

surgery or radiation exposure which makes reproduction impossible	surgery or radiation exposure to prevent reproduction done by doctor or medical termination of pregnancy (abortion)

↓ Means / ↓ Means / ↓ Means

Prohibition	listen to opinions of other doctors about the necessity beforehand	prior notification

Procedure

Elective Application	Consensual Application	Compulsory Application
Said person with consent of spouse or parent Application by spouse or parent	Hospital director diagnosing and treating said person, superintendant of public health center, esp. designated doctor Consent of spouse or parent	When the bad traits are significant, when the spouse also has bad traits, or when consent cannot be obtained, but limited to eugenic surgery on the ill person

Attached documents

Certificate of health
Report concerning heredity
Doctor's certificate giving notice of sterilization

Ruling → **Regional Director** — examination report → **Regional Eugenics Examination Committee**

Petition administration for redress → **Minister of Public Welfare** — examination report → **Central Eugenics Examination Committee**

Perform Surgery ↓

By designated doctor at designated hospital — Eugenic surgery

Notification is obligatory when the spouse makes application for the person undergoing eugenic surgery

with eugenics began with the transcription of the Yomiuri commemorative lecture[1] given at the YMCA hall on November 8, 1913. Katō Hiroyuki (see Chūman 2004, 285), Nitobe Inazō and other prominent people gathered to hear Nagai's lecture entitled "Discussion of the Necessity for the Study of Racial Betterment—Eugenics,"[2] in which he claimed that the relatively new "study of race betterment" based on "experimental genetics"[3] was necessary to be able to realize the highest ideals. Although Japan had not yet carried out statistical studies,[4] he had "sufficient statistics of the spread of bad seed in the United States" and introduced the situation of sterilization in California and Indiana (*Yomiuri Shimbun* Nov. 17, 1913). Although there is no direct evidence about the source of the information, it can be conjectured that it might have come from sources like the *Eugenical News*[5] first published in 1913, from the First International Congress of Eugenics[6] held in London in 1912, from Charles Davenport's *Heredity in Relation to Eugenics*[7] which had been published in 1911, or other eugenic works from America and Germany.

We turn our attention now to the sources of authority and support for Nagai's eugenic thought. A letter from the Ezra S. Gosney,[8] president of the Human Betterment Foundation in California offers us some insight. In the letter which began, "Dear Dr. Nagai, We have recently heard with great interest that the Ministry of Home Affairs of your country has ordered a survey concerning a eugenic sterilization law..." were enclosed sterilization survey results from ones done in the United States up until January 1, 1933 (Nagai 1934, 72-76). A translation (Saitō Shigesaburō 1933) of the foundation's pamphlet, entitled "Human Sterilization,"[9] was included in the second volume of the *Minzoku eisei sōsho*,[10] published by the Japanese Society of Racial Hygiene. The Japanese "elite" of today who have experience traveling to Western countries, go with a stronger self-esteem than others. But as long as they are of the "yellow race,"[11] they cannot sweep away the "racial dilemma;"[12] they are mindful that the awareness that they cannot acquire approval from the West cannot be swept away. That is, when they compare themselves with European and American intellectuals, it can be said that sharing a similar set of values proves self-excellence. I do not believe Nagai was an exception. It is my interpretation that his devotion to a eugenic educational campaign came from a desire to respond to Gosney's "Dear Dr. Nagai."

A positive attitude toward the passage of a sterilization law was also shown by social workers and psychiatrists in the late 1930s. The Japan Mental Hygiene Association, the Association of Public and Substitute Mental Hospitals, and the Help Associations submitted a "Petition concerning the inauguration of mental illness measures"[13] (1936) to the Home Minister urging the establishment and expansion of

1. 読売記念講演会　2.「人種改善学ユーゼニックスの必要を論ず」　3. 実験遺伝学
4. 統計処理　5. ユーゼニカル・ニューズ　6. 第1回国際優生学会議
7. C. ダヴェンポート『優生学に関わる遺伝』　8. 米国人類改善財団会長ガスネー
9.「人間の断種」　10.『民族衛生叢書』　11. 黄色人種　12. 人種的ジレンマ
13. 精神病対策確立に関する陳情書

national mental hospitals and the passage of a "sterilization law." In addition, the Japan Society of Psychiatry and Neurology established an "Investigation Committee for Heredity"[1] (1938) for psychosis cases. In the midst of such trends, the "Race Eugenic Protection Act Proposal," which nationalistic politicians had presented to the Imperial Diet numerous times since 1935, was enacted in 1940 as a government bill—*Kokumin Yūseihō* [The National Eugenic Law].[2]

b) Arguments against the sterilization law

But Japanese psychiatrists did not necessarily develop a simple sterilization promotion theory. The First Congress of the Nationwide Public Mental Hospital Directors Congress (1938) agreed with the view that "it is very desirable to enact a law to carry out sterilization only when heredity is certain or when the application is made by the person in question or a member of the family." However, the Japan Society of Psychiatry and Neurology was inclined to an opposing view or a cautious view. In particular, Kaneko Junji continued to voice opposition to the move to establish the "Race Eugenic Protection Law," which centered around Nagai Hisomu (Tanabe 1981, 875-883).

Yomiuri Shimbun published Kaneko's dissenting opinion along with an explanation of the situation:

> Since several years earlier when Dr. Nagai Hisomu and others began a movement to establish a "sterilization law," opponents said that from the standpoint of a criminal psychiatrist the "sterilization law" was an idealistic theory which would bring the nation to ruin. Among those taking a position of absolute opposition were Dr. Kaneko Junji of the Metropolitan Police Department's Medical Affairs Division[3] and Dr. Kikuchi Jinichi, sterilization medical examiner for the Tokyo District Court[4] .... In view of the fact that there were unexpectedly strong dissenting opinions among the experts in the field of psychiatry, the second committee meeting was postponed indefinitely based on the opinion of the Ministry of Health and Welfare and the committee in order to relieve friction as much as possible on every level concerning the law at hand, to carry out work harmoniously, and to plan how to soften the opposition (*Yomiuri Shimbun* evening edition, May 13, 1938).

In Nagai's rebuttal, "Opposition to the Opposition to the Sterilization Law,"[5] he asserted that "in order to make the fundamental spirit of the sterilization law complete, it would surely have to be compulsory" (Nagai 1934, 46-47). He emphasized that "a nation shows the standard of life for its citizens by its authority. He argued back saying:

---

1. 精神病に関する遺伝調査委員会   2. 国民優生法   3. 警視庁医務課の金子準二博士
4. 東京地方裁判所断種鑑定医菊池甚一博士   5. 永井潜「断種法に対する反対の反対」

"It is only for national security and happiness that as the populace lives its social life personal convenience of the individual is suppressed. In this sense, national societal interests must have first priority in the face of the law; the individual must come second." In addition, based on numerous data from Gosney and Popenoe, he asserted that it is clear that what is unfavorable to the one operated on, is to show kindness to the many. On the contrary, neglecting it to carry it out is "cruel."[1] Moreover, Nakatani cited the weakness of the legal force of the law,[2] the negative attitude of psychiatrists on site,[3] and the difficulty of systematic treatment due to the limited number of beds in mental hospitals as the reasons for the number of operations carried out being few in comparison to those in Germany (Nakatani 2000, 60).

c) Nagai Hisomu's disciples

It would not be an overstatement to say that the remarks of a Tokyo University doctor of medicine were enough to cause media reports about eugenics to run reckless. In particular, it can be said that Nagai Hisomu's "Yomiuri Commemorative Lecture" of November 8, 1913 for the 40th anniversary of publication was definitive. Based on "experimental genetics," "the study of race betterment—eugenics," while developing a new area of study, at the same time, "accepts that unfortunately just as various kinds of weeds grow rampant,[4] bad persons are likely to increase. ... If we do not pick out those with good genetic characteristics and eliminate those with bad ones,[5] we cannot attain our purpose. ... We have to eliminate from the world, those with mental illness, tuberculosis,[6] or family lines with other physical disabilities.[7] ... To do so, a law is necessary." Such comments by a 39-year old Tokyo Imperial University doctor of medicine[8] must have caused a considerable sensation. In his academic, fluent manner of talking, which, on occasion, reveals the "darkness" of human society[9] just as it is, we can make out Nagai's vividly revealed two-sidedness of "light and darkness." And it would be no exaggeration to say that this lecture would direct the course that Nagai would later follow. In other words, the discourse of 39 year old Nagai was not different at all from the 61 year old who reported in December 1936 that "The Sterilization Law Finally to the Diet." "If the Japanese nation hopes for eternal prosperity, the weeds that overrun the nation's flower garden must be pulled out by the roots through sterilization surgery"[10] (*Yomiuri Shimbun* morning edition December 12, 1936).

We turn our attention now to Teruoka Gitō,[11] who contributed to the establishment of the Ōhara Social Problems Institute (1919)[12] and studied at Tokyo University under Nagai Hisomu, Ōsawa Kenji,[13] Fujikawa Yū.[14] He can be called a pioneer in the study of women's issues and women's labor. Besides continuing his postgraduate research under Nagai, he was given the responsibility for a survey for the Metropolitan Police

1. 残忍　　2. 法の強制力の弱さ　　3. 現場の精神科医が消極的　　4. 雑草は能く蔓る
5. 良い遺伝物質を選って悪い物質を排除　　6. 精神病や結核　　7. 不具になる傾倒
8. 東京大学医学博士の言説　　9. 人間社会の「闇」
10.「民族の花園を荒す雑草は断種手術によって根こそぎに刈取る」　　11. 暉峻義等
12. 大原社会問題研究所　　13. 大澤謙二　　14. 富士川遊

Department and the Home Ministry. Combining medicine and social science, his survey of Tokyo's Honjo slum became a leading-edge study of a slum area in the field of social hygiene research.[1] Teruoka was employed as a "medical specialist" in the Ōhara Social Problems Institute and employed researchers like Ishikawa Tomoyoshi[2] (from Nagai's laboratory), Yagi Takatsugu[3] (from the Kitasato Institute), and Kirihara Shigemi[4] (on Fujikawa's recommendation), laying the groundwork for the Labor Science Institute. In Teruoka's book *Shakai eisei gaku*[5] [Study of social hygiene], six topics are given as social hygiene study methods and as an auxiliary science: statistical methods, anthropological biometry, economics, jurisprudence, psychology, race hygiene (population and eugenics).[6] These six topics are similar to the content outline of the *Shakai eisei nenkan* [Social hygiene yearbook][7] which Teruoka edited from May 1920 until 1952. For example, "sex hygiene,"[8] "heredity and constitution,"[9] and "racial hygiene"[10] are included in the twenty-five categories of documentary records. One can also catch a glimpse of information concerning eugenics and racial system (sterilization and miscegenation prohibition laws).

The questions for researchers of history are why at a set time in history certain systems, institutions, and systems of logic appeared or why the people living in that era thought to make such systems, institutions or systems of logic. Closing in on answers to these questions from historical documents is the real attraction of studying history.

Facts about the origin of eugenics in modern Japan[11] can be gained from going back to Nagai Hisomu's enlightenment activities and discourse.[12] Amid the voices of opposition and caution concerning the "sterilization law," the nation of that day demanded[13] that such a law be implemented. Nagai was just one who played a leading role in accomplishing its implementation. As long as one is in university post, one often runs up against the problem of "research or teaching." At such times the Humboldt principle[14] can be given as a reference: "Good researchers can become good educators. Good educators can at the same time become good researchers. They can carry out good research and communicate their results in education" (Arima 2000, 22-23). Both research and education are demanded from professors. As professor of physiology, Nagai was unable to accomplish either duty.

4. Eugenic Ideas in Postwar Health and Education and the Decline of Eugenics

In the 1960 government guidelines for teaching on the high school level,[15] "health of mothers and children,"[16] family planning,[17] and national eugenics"[18] were included in the guidance items. In 1970, "marriage and eugenics"[19] was one of the guidance items.

1. 社会衛生研究   2. 石川知福   3. 八木高次   4. 桐原葆見   5. 暉峻義等『社会衛生学』
6. 民族衛生（人口と優生）   7. 暉峻『社会衛生年鑑』   8. 「性の衛生」   9. 「遺伝及び体質」
10. 「人種衛生」   11. 近代日本における優生学の由来   12. 永井潜の啓蒙活動と言説
13. 当時の国家が要求   14. フンボルト理念   15. 高等学校学習指導要領   16. 母子衛生
17. 家族計画   18. 国民優生   19. 結婚と優生

However, it can be said that in educational circles, including the Ministry of Education, this way of thinking was already firmly established.

Also in textbooks the Eugenic Protection Act was given as the legal basis:

> To prevent passing on particularly bad hereditary ailments[1] in cases where there is a hereditary disease, such as schizophrenia,[2] manic-depressive psychosis,[3] total color blindness,[4] hemophilia,[5] hereditary deformities,[6] or in cases where the mother's life is in danger from childbirth, it has become possible to perform a eugenic operation or an induced abortion.[7] ... In the case where both family lines have hereditary defects or illness, it is preferable to avoid marriage all together. If unhealthy offspring are born, it leads to misfortune not only for the family, but for society as well. Such people should not leave behind descendants (Monbushō 1971, 1976, 1977).

After having specified such cases, the need for investigating family backgrounds[8] from the standpoint of eugenic marriage was emphasized.

However, the next revision of teaching guidelines included the following:

> National eugenics has been so strongly emphasized that there has been a tendency to violate the human rights of people who are physically or mentally handicapped,[9] and it has been pointed out that there is a social trend[10] to look down on the lives of children born with disabilities. Therefore, there is a growing inclination to reevaluate the Eugenic Protection Law.

The influence of eugenics began to decline, and, from 1978, items concerning eugenics were deleted. After that, the printed contents of textbooks gradually began to change.

The social background for this reversal was a movement opposing amniocentesis by the "*Aoi Shiba no Kai*"[11] 〔literally, the blue grass group〕, a group of people with cerebral palsy, and the strong criticism of the state's imposition of eugenic thought on its citizens. The result was a movement calling for the abolition of the Eugenic Protection Law.[12] In 1972, a revised Eugenic Protection Law was proposed, which included the following points:

1) the deletion of the economic reason for abortion and the addition of a mental reason,
2) the formation of a clause for selective abortion of a fetus with severe disabilities,

---

1. 悪質な遺伝性疾患　　2. 精神分裂病　　3. そううつ病　　4. 全色盲　　5. 血友病
6. 遺伝性奇形　　7. 優生手術や人工妊娠中絶　　8. 家系調査の必要性
9. 身体的精神的に障害をもつ人々の人権　　10. 社会的風潮
11. 「青い芝の会」の羊水検査反対運動　　12. 優生保護法撤廃を求める運動

3) the introduction of a guideline about the duties of the eugenic protection counselor, which includes instruction concerning a suitable age for the birth of the first child.

The proposed revisions of this law triggered the expansion of the activities of the "*Aoi Shiba no Kai.*" The revised bill was tabled and finally rejected.

The Eugenic Protection Law[1] was amended in 1996 to become the Maternal Protection Law. Three years later (1999), the high school curriculum was revised and the textbook content changed as follows:

> At the time of marriage, it is advisable to make sure of one another's health by such means as health examinations.[2]
> There is thought to be an appropriate age period for pregnancy and childbirth.[3]
> Family planning should proceed on the basis of a desire that every child be a child whose birth is eagerly awaited.
> Family planning is done mainly by birth control. For couples who want to get pregnant but cannot, there are medical treatments like the use of hormones to induce ovulation, artificial insemination,[4] and in vitro fertilization.[5]
> Even if pregnancy occurs when the birth of child is not wanted, surgery can be done on the fetus and placenta or medicine taken to discharge the fetus from the mother's body in what is called artificial abortion. In our country, according to the Maternal Protection Law, this is permitted under certain conditions. However, it should be noted that an artificial abortion takes away the life of the fetus, and an abortion without much thought is also problematic from the standpoint of respect for human life" (High school health and physical education, Hitotsubashi Publishers, 2002).

"At the time of marriage, it is advisable to make sure of one another's health..." Reading between the lines of these words from the textbook, I cannot help but be concerned that a national eugenic viewpoint is still firmly in place, conveying the idea of superior national traits and the intent of state policy[6] to demand eugenic marriages[7] and investigation of family lineages.[8]

Concluding Remarks

Nowadays, the problem of finding an appropriate way of policy-making for

---

1. 母体保護法　2. 健康診断　3. 妊娠・出産に適齢期　4. 人工受精　5. 体外受精
6. 国家政策の意図　7. 優生結婚　8. 家系調査

bioethical decisions is more and more difficult to solve. It is very important to find a common agreement on bioethical policy, especially in Japan, where it has been pointed out that there are only two extreme positions—"opposition to risk and social consensus."[1]

In the period before World War II, Japanese health administration was characterized by an extreme centralization of authority. The national management of human resources[2] was was carried out by hygiene administration of the police[3] under a system of surveillance and exposure,[4] disinfection and exclusion,[5] detention and segregation[6] implemented by the leadership of the Home Ministry. Therefore, the original framework was characterized by social discrimination and exclusion.

The hygiene administration drew a line of discrimination between the "clean" and the "filthy"[7] and aimed to eliminate the poor who had limited hygienic knowledge. On the other hand, eugenic thought aimed to discriminate, suppress, and exclude the inferior and hideous people. That is to say, the hygiene administration and eugenic thought had very similar stances toward the weak in society.

The enactment of the Eugenic Protection Law as well as its forerunner, the National Eugenics Law, was implemented under the leadership of eugenic advocates, that is, the elites in the academic world from the Meiji period. This fact is a well-known truth. It seems that what was at work to manipulate their arrogant, contemptuous, degrading valuation of the socially disadvantaged[8] was nothing more than their own inferiority complex. Many people were excluded from society or had their lives irreparably damaged by the spread of eugenic thought without adequate scientific evidence.[9] For this the leaders of eugenics in Japan bear a great responsibility. The blame and responsibility for this lie at the feet of the leaders of eugenics in Japan. [10]

Notes

*1 Tokyo University Library, Exposition Materials, Digital display: "Hakurankai kara mieru mono" ［博覧会から見えるもの What can be seen from exhibitions］. At the 1907 Louisiana Purchase International Exposition in St. Louis, Ainu people from Hokkaido were put on display in the Anthropology Department Ethnology Section. A photograph shows seven adults and two children (Yoshida 1999, 155; see also Vanstone 1993, 87).

*2 At the 5th Domestic Industrial Exhibition held in Osaka in 1903, a show booth called the "Anthropology Pavilion" was set up where various Asian ethnic groups were put "on display." This show became an issue in newspaper reports.

*3 In this volume is an aerial view of the Red Cross Society and central hospital from 1886 (Meiji 19) on page 60, the hospital in 1892 on page 207, an undated picture of an exhibit of a collection of valuable atomic bomb materials on page 32, and a picture of a "feebleminded

1. 慎重論と社会的合意論　　2. 人的資源の国家管理　　3. 警察の衛生行政
4. 監視と摘発　　5. 消毒と排除　　6. 収容と隔離　　7. きれいと不潔　　8. 社会的弱者
9. 十分な証拠を伴わない科学・技術と社会に関する言説
10. 日本における優生学提唱者の社会的責任

child with the fate of a halted mental development" on page 10. From these pictures and many others, one can visually grasp the activities of the Red Cross.

*4 This translation is from Jennifer Robertson (2002, 12). *Undō* can be translated both as exercise and movement.

*5 He is a different individual from postwar Prime Minister Yoshida Shigeru.

References

Arima Akito ［有馬朗人］, ed. 2000. *Kenkyūsha* ［研究者 Scholar］. Tokyo: Tokyo Tosho.

Chūman Mitsuko ［中馬充子］. 2004. "Kindai Nippon no Yūseishisō to kokka hokenseisaku" ［近代日本の優生思想と国家保健政策 Modern Japan's eugenic thought and national insurance policy］ in *Seimei no Rinri* ［生命の倫理 Ethics of Life］, Yamazaki Kiyoko ［山崎喜代子］, ed. Fukuoka: Kyushu Daigaku Shuppankai.

Fujino Yutaka ［藤野豊］. 1998. *Nippon fashizumu to yūseishisō* ［日本ファシズムと優生思想 Japanese fascism and eugenic thought］. Kyoto: Kamogawa Shuppan.

Fujime Yuki ［藤目ゆき］. 1997. *Sei no rekishigaku* ［性の歴史学 Historical science of sex］. Fuji Shuppan.

Gotō Ryūkichi ［後藤龍吉］. 1924～43. *Yūzenikkusu* ［ユーゼニックス Eugenics］（later *Yūseigaku* ［優生学］. Nippon Yuseigaku Kyokai. (Reprint 2013 Fuji Shuppan.).

Hirota Masaki ［ひろたまさき］. 1998. *Sabetsu no shisen — Kindai Nippon no Ishikikōzō* ［差別の視線―近代日本の意識構造］ Tokyo: Yoshikawa Kobunkan.

Horiguchi Ryōichi ［堀口良一］. 2000. *Sei to shi no shakaishi* ［生と死の社会史］. Yokohama: Shumpusha.

Hozumi Shigetoo ［穂積重遠］. 1941. *Kekkonkun* ［結婚訓］ Tokyo: Chuokoronsha.

Ikeda Shigenori ［池田林儀］. 1926~1930. *Yūsei Undō* ［優生運動 Eugenics exercise/movement］. Nippon Yusei Undo Kyokai.

Japan Red Cross ［日本赤十字］. 1928. *Sankōkan hō* ［参考館報 Archive Bulletin］, Third issue. Nippon Sekijujisha.

Japan Red Cross Society ［日本赤十字社］. 1955. *Nippon no Sekijūji* ［日本の赤十字 Japan's Red Cross］. Tokyo: Nippon Sekijujisha.

Katō Hiroshi ［加藤博史］. 1996. *Fukushiteki ningenkan no shakaishi—yūseishisō to hikō/seishinbyō wo tōshite* ［福祉的人間観の社会史―優生思想と非行・精神病を通して A social history of a humanitarian view of mankind: Delinquency and mental disease as seen in eugenic thought］ Kyoto: Koyo Shobo.

Kobashi Ichita ［小橋一太］. 1926. "Eisei shisō no fukyū" ［衛生思想の普及 Spread of hygienic thought］ in *Dai Nippon shiritsu eiseikai zasshi* ［大日本私立衛生会雑誌 Greater Japan Private Hygiene Association magazine］ 352 (Aug. 25), 481-477.

Kōseishō Yobōkyoku ［厚生省豫防局］. 1941. *Kokumin yusei zukai* ［國民優生図解 National eugenics illustrations］ (79 pages, available at the National Diet Library). Tokyo: Koseisho.

Monbusho (Kenteizumi Kyōkasho) ［文部省検定済教科書］. 1971, 1977. *Hokentaiiku* ［保健体育 Health and physical education］. Tokyo: Hitotsubashi Shuppan.

———. 1976. *Hyō-jun Kōtōhokentaiiku* ［標準高等保健体育 Standard High school health and physical education］. Tokyo: Kodansha.

Nagai Hisomu ［永井潜］. 1934. "Jinrui kaizen zaidan to sono soritsusha Gasunē " ［人類改善財團と其の創立者ガスネー］ in *Minzoku eisei* ［民族衛生］ 3, 72-76.

———. 1934. "Danshuhō ni taisuru hantai no hantai" ［斷種法に對する反對の反對 Opposition to the opposition to the sterilization law］ in *Minzoku eisei* ［民族衛生］ 3, 46-47.

Nagayo Sensai ［長與專齋］. 1884. "Kon'in heigairon" ［婚姻弊害論 Discussion of Marriage Abuse］ in *Dai Nippon shiritsu eiseikai zasshi* ［大日本私立衛生會雜誌 Greater Japan private hygiene association magazine］ 11 (1884), 1.

———. 1894. "Hakurankai no junbi" ［博覽會の準備 Preparations for the Exhibition］ in *Dai Nippon shiritsu eiseikai zasshi* ［大日本私立衛生會雜誌 Greater Japan private hygiene association magazine］ 132 (May 26, 1894), 421-439.

Nakatani Yōji ［中谷陽二］. 2000. *Senzen no Nihon ni okeru danshuhō wo meguru ronsō*, ［戦前の日本における断種法をめぐる論争 A look at the controversy concerning a sterilization law in prewar Japan］. in *Seishin igakushi kenkyū* ［精神医学史研究 Japanese journal of history of psychiatry］ 3, 60.

Ogata Masakiyo ［緒方正清］. 1907. *Fujin no kateieisei*. ［婦人の家庭衛生 Women's home hygiene］. Tokyo: Maruzen.

Oka Asajirō ［丘浅次郎］. 1911. "Minshu kaizengaku no jissai kachi" ［民種改善学の実際価値 The real value of ethnic betterment study］ (7:5)

Ono Yoshirō ［小野芳朗］. 1997. *Seiketsu no kindai* ［清潔の近代 Sanitary modern era］. Tokyo: Kodansha.

Robertson, Jennifer. 2002. "Blood Talks: Eugenic Modernity and the Creation of New Japanese" in *History and Anthropology* 13 :3, 191–216.

Sakanishi Tomohide ［坂西友秀］. 2005. *Kindai Nippon ni okeru jinshu/minzoku sutereotaipu to henken no keiseikatei* ［近代日本における人種・民族ステレオタイプと偏見の形成過程 The formation process of racial and ethnic stereotypes and prejudice］. Tokyo: Taga Shuppan.

Shimada Utako ［下田歌子］. 1906. *Jyoshi no eisei* ［女子の衛生 Female hygiene］. Tokyo: Fuzanbo.

Starr, Frederick. 1904. *The Ainu Group*. Chicago: Open Court Publishing Co. (Digital copy available at Cornell University Library 〈http://www.archive.org/details/cu31924080785441〉).

Tanabe Toshio ［田辺子男］. 1981. "Nihon no seishin igaku 100 nen wo kizuita hitobito" ［日本の精神医学 100 年を築いた人々 The people who built 100 years psychiatry in Japan］ in *Rinshō seishin igaku* ［臨床精神医学 Clinical psychiatry］ 10, 875-883.

Dai Nippon shiritsu eiseikai ［大日本私立衛生会］. *Dai Nippon shiritsu eiseikai zasshi* ［大日本私立衛生會雑誌 Greater Japan private hygiene association journal］ 132 (May 26, 1894), 469-574.

Takeda Hiroko. 2005. *The Political Economy of Reproduction in Japan: Between Nation-state and Everyday Life.* London: Routledge Curzon.

Tanaka Satoshi ［田中聡］. 1994. *Eiseitenrankai no yokubō* ［衛生展覧会の欲望 The desire of the public health exhibition］. Tokyo: Seikyusha.

Tanaka Yoshimaro ［田中義麿］. 1924. *Ningen honshitsu no kaizen ga kyūmu* ［人間本質の改善が急務 The betterment of human physical qualities is urgent］ ［医海及人間］ 2-3. Nagoya: Ikaioyobi Ningensha.

——. 1925. *Yūseigaku kara mita hainichimondai* ［優生学から見た排日問題 Looking at the anti-Japanese problem from eugenics］ *Yūseigaku* ［優生学 Eugenics］.

Tezuka Yoshiaki ［手塚義明］. 1942. *Sekijūji Dokuhon* ［赤十字読本 Red Cross Reader］. Tokyo: Japan Red Cross Society.

Unno Yukinori ［海野幸徳］. 1910. *Nippon jinshu kaizōron* ［日本人種改造論 On remodeling the Japanese Race］. Tokyo: Fuzanbo.

——. 1911. *Kōkokusaku to shite no jinshu kaizō* ［興国策としての人種改造 Race remodeling as a national policy］. Tokyo: Hakubunkan.

Vanstone, James W. 1993. "The Ainu Group at the Louisiana Purchase Exposition 1904" in *Arctic Anthropology* 30:2, 77-91.

Yamamoto Senji ［山本宣治］. 1925. *Sanji chōsetsu hyōron* ［産児調節評論 Birth Control Review］.

Yoshida Mitsukuni ［吉田光邦］. 1999. *Zusetsu bankoku tenrankaishi 1851-1942* ［図説万国博覧会史 1851-1942 Illustrated history of International Expositions 1851-1942］. Kyoto: Shibunkaku Shuppan.

Chapter 8 — Eugenics and Minorities

Fujino Yutaka

In a previous discussion of the relationship between eugenics and fascism[1] (Fujino 1998a), I noted that that sterilization laws[2] were enacted not only in Nazi era Germany and fascist era Japan, but also in America and Scandinavia, and that the Eugenic Protection Law[3] was enacted in postwar Japan. I came under criticism for over-emphasizing the ties between eugenics and fascism. However, this argument was based on the idea that eugenic policy was limited to sterilization laws only. Eugenics, as the name implies, promotes genetically well-born offspring,[4] but in reality, it seeks to prevent those considered to be genetically "inferior"[5] from bearing offspring. Of course, sterilization laws are not just carried out by fascist nations, but such nations not only implement sterilization laws, they also force their *not* genetically "inferior," healthy citizens to build up their physical strength. Thus the policies for healthy citizens and negative eugenic policies are two sides of the same coin and, as I see it, characteristics of a fascist nation.

Later, in answer to my critics, I discussed the campaigns to prevent the contagion of tuberculosis and venereal disease, the public health movement to use leisure time to discipline the mind and body, and the policy of seeking to increase the physical strength of soldiers from mountain villages where there were no medical facilities. I pointed out the fact that during the fascist era, Japan used the sterilization law to prevent the birth of "inferior persons" and, at the same time, forced those considered *not* inferior to maintain their health (Fujino 2003a, 2003b). In addition, I made clear the fact that, as the course of the war took a turn for the worse, the standards for soldiers were lowered and the "inferior" mentally disabled were drafted and under the illusion of pseudo-equality were sent to the battlefields. There were even plans to organize the quarantined Hansen's disease patients into "leprosy relief" volunteer corps and send them to battlefields. While being excluded from society, they were, at the same time, being included in the strategy for war mobilization[6] (Fujino 1993, 277-279). This side of eugenics under fascism should also not be forgotten.

1. ファシズム   2. 断種法   3. 優生保護法   4. 遺伝的に優秀な子孫
5. 遺伝的に「劣等」   6. 戦争動員

Meanwhile, because misinformation that I view eugenics as peculiar to fascism has been widely publicized and in protest thereof, I have continued my study of the treatment of minorities, especially the treatment of Hansen's disease patients. These minorities were judged to be "inferior" by eugenics, and this judgment not limited to the fascist era. This chapter will be based on my previous research and will examine how eugenic thought justified discrimination against minorities

1. Hansen's Disease Patients

Well-known even overseas, modern Japanese Christian leader Kagawa Toyohiko[1] served not only as a pastor, but also tackled various social problems and social enterprises. He was deeply involved in the labor movement, the peasant movement, and the *buraku*[*1] liberation movement, as well as being a pioneer in the "Mission to Lepers" movement for Hansen's disease patients. In particular, through his evangelistic efforts from 1909 involving the impoverished people of the Shinkawa slum adjoining Kobe's discriminated community area, Kagawa made a big impact on social problems.

In 1915 in the midst of World War I, Kagawa published *Hinmin Shinri no Kenkyū*[2] [The Study of the Psychology of the Poor] based on his experiences in Shinkawa. In this book describing his findings about the causes of the poverty and its solution, Kagawa cited alcohol addiction[3] and "unhappy marriages."[4] As specific examples of the latter, he listed "early marriages, adultery, marriages of unfit persons,"[*2] consanguineous marriages, imprudent marriages, and other lustful sexual relations, as are often seen in impoverished slums. Here he emphasized the marriage of the "unfit."

As can be seen in his comment that "idiots, the retarded, and the mentally ill who were already married and in their prime were continuing to produce a lower race," Kagawa first of all meant by "unfit" those who have mental disabilities or mental disorders. But he did not stop there. He counted criminals among the unfit because criminality was considered to be inherited. The *burakumin* were included as well because there were many criminals among them. He referred to them as "Japan's degenerate race," "the criminal race of Imperial Japan," and "Japan's prostitute race."

Moreover, by saying that "since nymphomania[5] is likely due to the heredity of alcoholics and syphilis patients" many poor people are born from "nymphomaniacs," alcoholics and syphilis patients were included in the numbers of "unfit" too. All such "unfit" could be wiped out and the problem of poverty solved by "race improvement."[6]

What Kagawa meant here by "race improvement" is sterilization. The eugenic policy of sterilizing the "unfit" and cutting off their offspring was seen by Kagawa to be

---

1. 賀川豊彦　2.『貧民心理の研究』　3. アルコール依存症　4.「不幸なる結婚」
5. 色情狂　6.「人種改良」

an effective solution for the problem of poverty. Later, when he went so far as to seek the "Law for Race Improvement" for alcoholics and syphilitics who lack organizational knowledge, it is apparent that Kagawa's understanding of the problem of poverty was based on eugenics (Kagawa 1926).

At the time Kagawa was writing *Study of the Psychology of the Poor*, Tokyo Imperial University physiology professor Nagai Hisomu,[1] social work researcher Unno Yukinori,[2] technician of the Home Ministry Department of Public Health Ujihara Sukezō,[3] and others were calling for the need to sterilize the "unfit" and started debate concerning eugenic policy. For them, by implementing sterilization, Japan could, both in terms of quantity and quality of population, gain an advantage over Europe and America after World War I. Also at this time, several American states had already begun sterilization under state laws. And at this time, the Director of the Hansen's disease sanatorium, the Zensei Hospital,[4] Mitsuda Kensuke,[5] played a role in promoting a policy of absolute segregation for life for all Hansen's disease patients. It was also in 1915, the year *Study of the Psychology of the Poor* was published, that Mitsuda, with surgery conducted on a male patient, began implementing sterilization of patients. I'll address this issue in greater detail in the next chapter.

Nagai, his colleagues, and Kagawa all held similar opinions. And, from the perspective of eugenic policy, a focus on leprosy evolved. In 1927 Kagawa lamented "We, as a superior nation, are unable to stand up to Caucasians proudly," one of the reasons being the increasing number of lepers (Kagawa, 1927a). Based on eugenic thought, in order to raise the intelligence, mental, and physical strength to a level where Japanese could compete with Caucasians as a "superior race," Kagawa sought to wipe out Hansen's disease patients. "As to why I nag about the problem of leprosy, it is to raise the social efficiency of the nation" (Kagawa, 1927b). As seen in this declaration, the reason why Kagawa focused on Hansen's disease came as an outgrowth of his eugenic ideas (see Fujino 2011).

2. *Burakumin*

However, ridding the nation of defective people was not an idea unique to Kagawa. According to prejudice toward the *hisabetsuburaku* people at that time, it was thought that, as a result of avoiding marriage with outsiders and repeated consanguineous marriages, hereditary Hansen's disease and physical disabilities were widespread, or that reproductive functions were abnormal (see Fujino 1998a, 399-405). In particular, concerning Hansen's disease, the state of affairs gave rise to a nationwide investigation of

---

1. 永井潜   2. 海野幸徳   3. 氏原佐蔵   4. 全生病院   5. 光田健輔

the areas where *burakumin* lived. Conducted in 1916 by Mitsuda Kensuke, director of the Hansen's disease sanatorium Zensei Hospital, this investigation was based on the prejudice that Hansen's disease often appeared among the *burakumin* (see Fujino 2006, chapter 1). At that time, just as the terms "special village" (different from the ordinary *tokushuburaku*[1]) and "special kind of village" (*tokushuburaku*[2]) were used (see Fujino 1994), the perception that the *burakumin* were genetically "inferior" spread throughout society and became the justification for avoiding intermarriage with them (see Fujino 1999).

3. Ainu

In addition, after the Meiji Restoration, the Ainu people, "a perishing race,"[3] were considered a suitable subject for eugenic research. The purpose of this research was to ask why the Ainu were dying out, medically clarify the reasons, and ensure that Japanese did not follow the same path.

Investigation of the Ainu was begun in the summer of 1932 by the Japan Society of Race Hygiene,[4] which was at the forefront of the push to implement eugenic policy. Member of the board of directors, Koya Yoshio[5] (Chiba Medical University), made an inspection tour and conducted a census of the Ainu. Afterwards, research was begun "on the important matters of the physical condition of the vanishing race of the Ainu, the reasons for their decline, and the problem of inter-marriage—matters which needed to be presented at academic meetings around the world." It was expected that the solution for the cause of this crisis found in these investigations would be "reference material for the prosperous progress of our Yamato race" (*Hokkai Times* Aug. 27, 1933). Thus, in July 1934 the first survey was begun in the Hokkaido village of Hiratori in Saru County.[6] But prior to the entire survey, in late May, 131 complete skeletons were excavated from an Ainu cemetery in Yakumo City Yūrabbu Beach,[7] under the jurisdiction of the Oshima[8] subprefectural office, and measurements were conducted. Concerning this survey, the Japan Association of Race Hygiene praised its own work by saying: "the results of eugenics studies using living materials have repercussions for the future development evolution of our cultural people, serve as an object lesson, and cast a warning light" (*Minzoku eisei* 3:6 [Sept. 1934], 101-102). Hokkaido Imperial University Anatomy Department professor Kodama Sakuzaemon,[9] who excavated the tombs, said in defense that his action was not grave-robbing since it was done with the local Ainu people's approval. Moreover, a grave marker was erected and a memorial service was conducted afterwards in accordance with Ainu religious practices. People who, on the other hand,

1. 特殊部落　2. 特種部落　3. 『滅び行く民族』　4. 日本民族衛生学会
5. 古屋芳雄　6. 平取村沙流郡　7. 八雲町遊楽部浜　8. 渡島　9. 児玉作左衛門

opposed the excavation were regarded with disdain as "highly superstitious old folks" and "obstinate old timers" (Kodama, 1936). This view of scholars, with their pride as a "superior ethnic group," reveals their eugenic discrimination toward those they considered an "inferior ethnic group." Kodama and his colleagues regarded the Ainu as an ethnic group which was headed for extinction and as a subject for eugenic study. They opened Ainu tombs, carried away the buried remains and skeletons as specimens, and conducted various measurements of them in order to demonstrate their "inferiority" (Ueki 2008, 95-131; Fujino 1998a, 216-259).

4. Prostitutes

Prostitutes became yet another target of eugenics. The derogatory term, *shūgyōfu*[1] [lit. disgraceful work woman] by which they were referred, was not just a moral term, it also included a discriminatory eugenic view of them as the source of infection for sexual diseases and the main culprit for demeaning society.

With the Meiji Restoration, the *yūkaku*[2] [pleasure quarters] were renamed *kashizashiki*[3] [tatami rooms for hire]. In cities and prefectures "red-light districts" were demarcated by the police. A system of legal prostitution was established, and prostitutes were given a license that allowed them to work. However, in 1900 the Home Ministry's "Regulation for the Control of Prostitutes"[4] stipulated that prostitutes were to be over 18 years of age and to have regular mandatory medical checkups and, when necessary, treatment for venereal disease. As long as brothel keepers complied with the law, prostitution was permitted, and the accompanying human trafficking was condoned. In 1907 when the penal code was promulgated, human trafficking was not specified as a crime (Fujino 2012, 14-24). Thus, the prevention of the spread of sexual diseases became one reason for the support of legal prostitution. As the moniker used then, "hereditary syphilis,"[5] illustrates, emphasis was placed on contagion in the womb—the contagion of the fetus by the mother. In this respect, sexually transmitted disease was a subject of eugenic thought, and the health management of prostitutes was a part of eugenic policy.

Those who approved of brothel keepers and prostitutes claimed it was for the cause of the greater good, maintaining that legalized prostitution prevented the spread of venereal disease. Proponents for prohibition of public prostitution argued that the system only spread the contagion of sexual diseases. The basis of their argument was that men who visited prostitutes were infected by them, and they, in turn, infected their wives, who then infected their children. Thus, prostitution results in the birth of congenitally

1. 醜業婦　　2. 遊廓　　3. 貸座敷　　4. 「娼妓取締規則」　　5. 「遺伝性梅毒」

defective children. As is evident from this logic, eugenic thought existed even in the movement to abolish prostitution.

The Purity Society,[1] a nationwide prostitution prohibition group, featured a series on "Heredity and Environment" in their publication *Kakusei*[2] [The Purity]. The preface makes the following declaration:

> eugenics is the newest academic field. That is, from the standpoint of those who lecture on the morality of males and females in an attempt to reform society, the influence of heredity and environment needs to be clarified. Actively creating a superior environment and a superior race must be the mission of this society (*Kakusei* 8 Sept./Oct. 1918).

This logic is also evident in the 1920 campaign in the 42nd Imperial Diet Session by the *Shinfujin kyōkai*[3] [New Woman Association]. This association, founded by Hiratsuka Raichō[4] and Ichikawa Fusae,[5] presented their Marriage Restriction against Men with Venereal Disease petition[6] to the Diet. This campaign sought a law stating that marriage would be prohibited for men who had contracted *karyūbyō*[7] [red light district diseases]—sexually transmitted diseases. The rationalization for such a law was the

> protection of the women who would become their wives and at the same time protection of future children. It would strengthen the nation and improve the quality of the nation's people. It would also serve the good of the racial stock, which is the obligation of both men and women alike (Hiratsuka, 1920).

Later in 1927, a Venereal Disease Prevention Law[8] was promulgated seeking the same kind of measures to prevent infectious sexual diseases among unlicensed prostitutes as had been taken for licensed prostitutes. However, when soldiers began returning from China after the Sino-Japanese war, they brought back venereal diseases to all parts of the nation. In order to prevent the spread of infection, this law was revised to include not just unlicensed prostitutes, but was expanded to include all citizens. Here, the understanding of venereal disease as an issue of eugenic policy is illustrated.

This fact is closely connected with the installation of so-called "military comfort women."[9] The necessity and aim of putting "military comfort women" in place was seen as preventing rape of women nearby and raising the soldiers' morale. However, it was not limited to these reasons. Another reason was to prevent the soldiers from being infected by hiring a prostitute on the battlefield and spreading that infection upon their

1. 廓清会   2. 『廓清』   3. 新婦人協会   4. 平塚らいてう   5. 市川房江
6. 花柳病男子結婚制限法制定運動   7. 花柳病   8. 花柳病予防法   9. 従軍慰安婦

return to Japan. From a eugenic standpoint, it was deemed necessary to have "military comfort women" under army management, who were checked regularly for infection by a military doctor. It should be remembered that the eugenic idea of protecting the quality of a superior people provided the background for facilitating "military comfort women" (Fujino 1998b, 54-61).

In Conclusion

Eugenic thought is one of discrimination. It is as if under the logic of the academic evidence of genetics, discrimination is made on the basis of human differences, and then the ones who decide who is "inferior" and who is "superior" set out to "prove" it. Eugenic thought is not just held by governments. It was held by members of social movements, as seen in the ideas of their representatives—Kagawa Toyohiko, Hiratsuka Raichō and Ichikawa Fusae. Among those who promoted the passage of the postwar Eugenic Protection Law were many Japan Socialist Party[1] lawmakers. Eugenic thought before World War II provided the justification for building a strong military nation which could stand face to face with Western nations. After the war, eugenics was justified for building a cultural nation. Under the guise of science, discrimination against people who are deemed "inferior" is rationalized. At present, under the justification of medicine, called prenatal diagnosis,[2] society is ready to accept eugenic thought once again. We need to be aware that eugenic thought is discriminatory.

Notes

*1 *Buraku* (部落) refers to a hamlet, a community; *burakumin* (部落民) to people from certain communities who have been the targets of discrimination in Japanese society. Discrimination began in the Edo period (late 16th century to 17th century) under a hierarchical feudal caste system in which social class was inherited. These people, though not a separate ethnic group, were ostracized from the rest of society and were involved in occupations that were considered impure or tainted by death, such as executioners, undertakers, slaughterhouse workers, butchers, tanners, etc. Legally, this status ended with the Meiji Restoration in 1868, but social attitudes did not change with the law. *Burakumin* is the term most often used in English, but the term used most often now in Japanese is *hisabetsuburaku* (被差別部落) people— "discriminated community" people.

*2 The expression used by Kagawa is literally "person with bad qualities" [akushitsusha 悪質者] and refers to people considered to have bad genes. "Unfit," the most often used English expression, is used here.

1. 日本社会党   2. 出生前診断

References

Fujino Yutaka [藤野 豊]. 1993. *Nihon fashizumu to iryō—Hansenbyō wo meguru jisshōteki kenkyū* [日本ファシズムと医療―ハンセン病をめぐる実証的研究 Japanese facism and medical care—demonstrative study about Hansen's disease]. Tokyo : Iwanami Shoten.

———. 1994. "Hisabetsu buraku" [被差別部落 Discriminated-against community] in *Iwanami kōza Nihon tsūshi kindai 3* [岩波講座日本通史 近代 3 Iwanami lecture of the general history of Japan], 139-155. Tokyo: Iwanami Shoten.

———. 1998a. *Nihon fashizumu to yūseishisō* [日本ファシズムと優生思想 Japanese fascism and eugenic thought]. Kyoto: Kamogawa Shuppan.

———. 1998b. "Nihon fashizumu to seibyō" [日本ファシズムと性病 Japanese fascism and sexual diseases] in *Kikan sensō sekinin kenkyū* [季刊戦争責任研究 Study of War Responsibility Quarterly] 22 (Dec.), 54-61.

———. 1999, "Buraku mondai ni okeru kon'in kihi" [部落問題における婚姻忌避 Avoidance of marriage in the *buraku* problem] in *Gendai shisō* [現代思想 Present day thought] 27:2, 84-95.

———. 2000. *Kyōsei sareta kenkō—Nihon fashizumuka no seimei to shintai* [強制された健康―日本ファシズム下の生命と身体 Forced health—Life and body under Japanese fascism]. Tokyo: Yoshikawa Kobunkan.

———. 2001. *Sei no kokka kanri—baibaishun no kingendaishi* [性の国家管理―買売春の近現代史 The control of sex: Modern history of sexual exploitation]. Tokyo: Fuji Shuppan.

———. 2003. *Kōseishō no tanjō—iryō wa fashizumu wo ika ni suishin shita ka* [厚生省の誕生―医療はファシズムをいかに推進したか The birth of the Ministry of Health—how medical care supported fascism]. Kyoto: Kamogawa Shuppan.

———. 2006. *Hansen byō to sengo minshushugi—naze kakuri wa kyōsei sareta no ka* [ハンセン病と戦後民主主義―なぜ隔離は強化されたのか Hansen's disease and postwar democracy—why was segregation forced?]. Tokyo: Iwanami Shoten.

———. 2010a. *Senso to Hansenbyo* [戦争とハンセン病 War and Hansen's disease]. Tokyo: Yoshikawa Kobunkan.

———. 2010b. "Teikoku guntai to hogohei" [帝国軍隊と保護兵 The imperial army and the protection army] *Kikan sensō sekinin kenkyū* [季刊戦争責任研究 Study of War Responsibility Quarterly] 69 (Sept.), 2-13.

———. 2011. "Kagawa Toyohiko to 'Kyūrai' Undō" [賀川豊彦と「救癩」運動 Kagawa Toyohiko and the "Leprosy Relief movement"] in *Nihon Kirisutokyōshi ni okeru Kagawa Toyohiko—Sono shisō to Jissen* [日本キリスト教史における賀川豊彦―その思想と実践 Toyohiko Kagawa in Japanese Christian History: Thought and Application] ed. Kagawa Toyohiko Kinen Matsuzawa Shiryōkan. Shinkyo Shuppansha, 525-549.

———. 2012. *Sengo Nihon no jinshin baibai* [戦後日本の人身売買 Postwar Japan's human trafficking]. Tokyo: Otsuki Shoten.

Hiratsuka Raichō. 1920. "Karyūbyō danshi kekkonseigenhō seitei ni kansuru seigan undō" [花柳病男子結婚制限法制定に関する請願運動 Campaign to petition for marriage restriction against men with venereal disease] in *Josei dōmei* [女性同盟 Women's league], 1 (Oct.) in *Hiratsuka Raichō's Works* 3, 173-175, 177. Tokyo: Otsuki Shoten.

Kagawa Toyohiko [賀川豊彦]. 1915. *Hinmin Shinri no Kenkyū* [貧民心理の研究 Study of the Psychology of the Poor]. Tokyo: Keiseisha.

——. 1926. *Binbō wo sukuu Michi* [貧乏を救ふ道 Road to Redemption of Poverty] Gakujutsukoen Tsushinsha.

——. 1927a. "Shin Nihon no shōgen" [新日本の証言 The Testimony of New Japan] in *Hi no Hashira* [火の柱 Pillar of Fire] 12 (February) 1-2.

——. 1927b. "Shakai mondai to shite mitaru raibyō zetsumetsu undō" [社会問題として見たる癩病絶滅運動 The movement to totally eradicate leprosy as seen as a social problem] in *Hi no Hashira* [火の柱 Pillar of Fire] 6:3 (March), 9.

Kikuchi, Ichiro. 1997. "Hansen's disease in Japan: a brief history" in *International Journal of Dermatology* 36:8, 629-633.

Kodama Sakuzaemon [児玉作左衛門]. 1936. "Yakumo Yūrabbu ni okeru Ainu funbo iseki no hakkutsu" [八雲遊楽部に於けるアイヌ墳墓遺跡の発掘 The excavation of the ruins of Ainu graves in Yakumo Yūrabbu" in *Hokkaidō Teikoku Daigaku igakubu kaibōgaku kyōshitsu kenkyū hōkoku* [北海道帝国大学医学部解剖学教室研究報告 Report of Anatomy Studies of the Medical Department of Hokkaido Imperial University], 1 (Nov.), 2-3.

Reber, Emily A. Su-lan. 1999. "*Buraku mondai* in Japan: Historical and Modern Perspectives and Directions for the Future" in *Harvard Human Rights Journal*, 12 (Spring) 297~359.

Sato, Hajime [佐藤元]. 2003. " Politics of leprosy segregation in Japan—The emergence, transformation and abolition of the patient segregation policy" in *Social Science and Medicine* 56 (June), 2529-2539.

Ueki Tetsuya [植木哲也]. 2008. *Gakumon no bōryoku: Ainu bochi wa naze abakareta ka* [学問の暴力―アイヌ墓地はなぜあばかれたか Academic violence: why was the Ainu cemetery violated?]. Yokohama: Shumpusha.

Yoshimi, Yoshiaki [吉見義明]. 2000. *Comfort Women: Sexual Slavery in the Japanese Military during World War II*. Suzanne O'Brien, trans. New York: Columbia University Press.

Chapter 9

Eugenics and Hansen's Disease Patients

Fujino Yutaka

*I*n the previous chapter we looked at several minority groups who were targets of eugenic policy in Japan. Of these groups, Hansen's disease patients were subject to segregation and sterilization.[1] This chapter will address the question of why Hansen's disease patients, even though their disease was not hereditary, were targeted by sterilization laws.

The National Eugenic Law,[2] the sterilization law, was promulgated in 1940, and put in operation in April of the following year. The subjects of sterilization were the sick and handicapped whose condition was considered genetic, primarily the mentally disabled. Accordingly, sterilization was legally carried out from 1941, but actually from 1915 Hansen's disease patients were sterilized outside of the law. Under the Act on Leprosy Prevention,[3] promulgated in 1907, the state presented Hansen's disease not as a genetic disease, but as a frightening contagious disease, exaggerated its infectivity, and established an absolute segregation policy which subjected all patients to lifelong quarantine. In addition, this state policy which was revised in 1953 was consistent with the Act on Leprosy Prevention. However, on the other hand, sterilization was performed on Hansen's disease patients as if the disease were genetic. The question at hand is why Hansen's disease patients, who had been excessively publicized as contagious and driven into absolute isolation, were made the targets of sterilization. I will offer some answers in the paragraphs that follow.

1. Sterilization

The hospital where sterilizations were carried out in 1915 was the National Hansen's Disease Sanatorium Zensei Hospital[4] in Tokyo, whose director that year was Mitsuda Kensuke.[5] In Mitsuda's postwar memoir *Kaishun Byōshitsu*[6] (Mitsuda 1950a), he states that spouses, who were both lifelong segregated patients, requested not to have children through sterilization in exchange for being permitted to have marital relations

---

1. 断種   2. 国民優生学   3. らい予防法   4. 全生病院   5. 光田健輔
6. 『回春病室』

and that this request was granted on the basis of humanitarian consideration. The reasons why Hansen's disease patients should not bear children as given by Mitsuda are: infection of the child through contact, deterioration of the mother's condition during pregnancy or childbirth, bad influences on roommates due to the crying of the children, and the difficulty of raising children in segregation. These comments, however, come from after the war, when the Hansen's disease sanatorium patients' movement became active. The veracity of these comments cannot be taken at face value. In fact, doctors who specialized in Hansen's disease gave different reasons at their conferences. One of those reasons was the myth of a predisposition to Hansen's disease.

Mitsuda Kensuke was the doctor who initiated sterilization of Hansen's disease patients. Already in 1906, when he was the medical officer of the Tokyo City Orphanage Hospital, he had accepted the existence of "a body type susceptible to leprosy" (Mitsuda 1906), denied the perception of Hansen's disease as an inherited disease, and promoted a policy of segregation based on the hype touting its infectivity. From this it can be seen that the idea of a physical constitution in which the symptoms of Hansen's disease easily appeared and the possibility of inheriting such a tendency existed in the medical world. One person holding such a view was Suzue Kitasu.[1]

In April of 1931, Kumamoto Medical University Suzue Kitasu and his colleagues made a presentation entitled "The Essential Study of Leprosy" at the 21st annual meeting of the Japan Society of Pathology. In their attempt "to some degree probe into the true character of predisposition of leprosy and into its contagion," they presented their results of measuring twenty-nine skulls of Hansen's disease patients (Suzue and Nagase 1931).

2. Skeletal Specimens

Suzue, who graduated from Kyoto Imperial University Medical School in 1924 and afterwards continued study in the Department of Pathology, took a position at the Kumamoto University School of Medicine in 1927. There he procured the remains of patients from the National Hansen's Disease Sanatorium in Kyushu and constructed more than fifty skeletal specimens (Suzue 1951, 53-54). Suzue accepted the existence of a predisposition to developing Hansen's disease, thought that these characteristics would be evident in skeletal features, prepared the specimens, and conducted skull measurements.

This concept is similar to Kodama Sakuzaemon's[2] attempt to prove the "inferiority" of the Ainu people by excavating their tombs and removing bones from them—a concept based on eugenic thought. It should also be noted that it was Kiyono Kenji[3] who

1. 鈴江懐　　2. 児玉作左衛門　　3. 清野謙次

encouraged Suzue to research Hansen's disease. Suzue was under Kiyono's tutelage while studying in the Pathology Department of Kyoto Imperial University. (Kiyono is also known for instructing Ishii Shirō[1] and other members of Unit 731 of the Japanese Imperial Army.[2][*1]) From 1921, Kiyono was a professor in the Department of Microbiology of the Kyoto Imperial University's School of Medicine and was concurrently professor of pathology from 1924. He also had interests in archaeology and anthropology and conducted excavations of shell mounds. From measurements carried out on bones excavated from the Tsukumo shell mounds in Okayama prefecture, Kiyono set out to prove that there was no special resemblance of the Ainu people and Japanese of the Jōmon period. In order to do so, he traveled to Sakhalin in 1924, excavated Ainu tombs, digging up the skeletons of fifty-two bodies (Ueki 2008, 72-75). It can be surmised that Suzue's construction of skeletal specimens of Hansen's disease patients came from Kiyono's influence. Suzue thought that he would find some distinguishing features in the bones of Hansen's disease patients, but was unable to find any proof for his hypothesis. Without the support of the academic society, Suzue soon lost interest. His skeleton specimens were abandoned and destroyed in the war.[*2]

Even so, Suzue's research on the susceptibility of Hansen's disease was continued off and on thereafter. In 1941, Suzue summarized the history of research of the predisposition theory, in which he stated:

> In comparison to that of ten years ago, society's conventional wisdom concerning leprosy is certainly greater today. We will not be merely caught in infantile groundless fears, but will seriously face the problem of "leprosy and physical makeup" and apply the solemn scalpel of science (Suzue 1941).

From the context, the expression "infantile groundless fears" refers to the claim that one ought to refrain from discussing the relationship between Hansen's disease and a susceptible body type because it might cause a misunderstanding that Hansen's disease is a genetic disease. Suzue claimed that research of the relation between Hansen's disease and predisposition should be expanded, irrespective of such opinion.

However, as mentioned earlier, Suzue's attention moved away from the skeletons of patients. In 1943 Suzue reported on postmortem autopsies done in collaboration with Kikuchi Keifu-en[3] National Hansen's Disease Sanatorium director Miyazaki Matsuki.[4] Their research was based on the hearts of thirty-one patients of the sanatorium (Suzue 1943). At the end of his memoirs, Suzue wrote:

---

1. 石井四郎　2. 731部隊　3. 菊池恵風園　4. 宮崎松記

I had already found an allergic tissue reaction resulting in rheumatoid nodules in the leprous heart and in the beriberi heart. The connection of both of these conditions and the analysis of that connection present me a big challenge for the future (Suzue 1951, 55).

As these comments indicate, Suzue's later research was "leprosy allergy," namely elucidating the relation between Hansen's disease and allergic predisposition.

3. Physical Constitution

Suzue's research is emblematic of fact that research into the existence of a physical constitution susceptible to Hansen's disease was promoted where health care for Hansen's disease patients was provided. However, because argument about it would cause a misunderstanding that Hansen's disease is a genetic disease, and as a result, raise questions among the public about the policy of absolute segregation, prudence was deemed necessary. Around the same time, Suzue was discussing the relationship between Hansen's disease and physical constitution, the 4th General Meeting of the Japan Leprosy Society was held in March 1931. In this meeting Sotojima Hoyō-in[1] director Murata Masataka,[2] under the title *"Rai no idensetsu ni tai suru hihan"* [Criticism concerning the theory of leprosy inheritance], criticized the discussion of Hansen's disease related to predisposition and predisposition related to heredity. Murata's criticism was not made from an academic standpoint, but a political one based on the fear that such theories could give the wrong idea about Hansen's disease and genetic disease. In Suzue's words, this was an "infantile groundless fear." At that time, Ōshima sanatorium[3] director Kobayashi Wasaburō[4] countered the criticism with clinical examples, saying that even if Hansen's disease is a contagious malady, contagion is influenced by physical makeup (*Lepra* 2: 2 June 1931, 61-62). Even afterwards, study emphasizing the relationship of Hansen's disease and a body type predisposed to infection was continued. Hokubu Hoyōin[5] [Northern Therapy Center] director Nakajō Suketoshi[6] asserted that "in the case that Hansen's disease has a susceptibility factor it is that of contagion" (Nakajō 1934). Kuryū Rakusen-en[7] director Takashima Shigetaka[8] also pointed out "concerning the contraction of leprosy, one should consider a genetic predisposition factor" (Takashima 1939). And Zensei Hospital director Hayashi Yoshinobu, in a research presentation for the 13th General Meeting of the Japan Leprosy Society in entitled *"Oyako oyobi dōho rai kanja"* [Parent and child as well as fellow leprosy patients], accepted the heredity of a body type susceptible to Hansen's disease (Hayashi

---

1. 外島保養院   2. 村田正太   3. 大島療養所   4. 小林和三郎   5. 北部保養院
6. 中條資俊   7. 栗生楽泉園   8. 高島重孝

1940). As can be seen from the comments of these three directors who promoted absolute segregation, the opinion that there was a close relationship between Hansen's disease contagion and a body type predisposed to infection was held by no few people.

However, as is evident from Murata Masataka's comments, should such a fact be widely disclosed to the public, there was the possibility of losing the justification for absolute segregation policy. This stance that one's physical constitution affected the incidence of leprosy and thus necessitated a policy of absolute quarantine was not without criticism. The theory of Ogasawara Noboru[1] of the special research lab of the dermatology clinic attached to Kyoto Imperial University School of Medicine was reported on February 22, 1941 by the *Chūgai Nippō* [Domestic and Foreign Daily] with the titles "Leprosy is not Incurable" and "The Theory that Leprosy is Infectious is not entirely credible." In addition, the July 3 edition of the Osaka *Asahi Shimbun* reported: "Leprosy is not a contagious disease,[2] but a 'constitutional disease'[3]—a new theory from Kyoto." These reports resulted in fierce attacks on Ogasawara by doctors who promoted absolute segregation. At the 15th Annual Meeting of the Japan Leprosy Society held on November 15 and 16, moderator Murata went as far as suppressing Ogasawara's comments and gave a speech calling Ogasawara's theories mistaken.

However, on the other hand, on the day after the turbulent Leprosy Society Meeting the second "Joint Research of Leprosy"[4] committee meeting supported by the Ministry of Education Scientific Research Fund[5] was held at Osaka Imperial University School of Medicine. Participants at the meeting included Ogasawara, Mitsuda Kensuke, and other directors of sanatoria. The minutes of the meeting record the following:

> Up till now there has been a tendency to avoid the study of the relationship between leprosy and physical constitution. But as facts are facts, there is the need for thorough study. However, prudence must be exercised in reporting of the results of the study (Document of 2nd conference about Hansen's Disease by Scientific Research fund of Ministry of Education).

Thus they confirmed the necessity of researching whether there is a physical constitution that is susceptible to Hansen's disease and whether such a constitution is hereditary. There was also agreement that making the results of this research public required discretion. This put a restraint on Ogasawara, while at the same time giving his theories scientific recognition (see Fujino 2012). Here it becomes clear that an understanding of genetic predisposition was a reason for the forcible sterilization of Hansen's disease patients (see Fujino 2013).

1. 小笠原登　2. 伝染病　3.「体質病」　4.「癩ニ関スル協同研究」
5. 文部省科学研究費

4. Fetal Specimens[1]

However, this was not the sole reason for sterilizing Hansen's disease patients. Another was the theory that Hansen's disease was a sexually transmitted disease.[2] Based on this theory, leprosy bacilli breed in the testes and would be mixed in the semen of male patients. Females would be infected during sexual intercourse. The bacillus would then, in turn, infect the fetus through the placenta. This was the kind of logic on which Mitsuda Kensuke based the need for sterilization—the possibility of infection through the placenta and semen (Mistuda 1936). Nojima Taiji[3] also insisted that in order to prevent the "reproductive contagion"[4] of Hansen's disease, "the most important element of leprosy policies is an abortion law or a contraception law for leprosy patients" (Nojima 1932). The issue here is whether or not there is placental infection. If this is accepted, then Hansen's disease becomes a hereditary disease—passed from mother to child—where the fetus is born with congenital Hansen's disease. From a eugenic point of view, whether or not there is placental infection of Hansen's disease became an important topic of research. And, as an extension of this, the issue of constructing specimens of fetuses comes to the surface.

According to the "Verification Committee Concerning Hansen's Disease Problem Final Report Supplement : Report on survey of fetal specimens"[5] (2005), during the investigation of all of the national Hansen's disease sanatoria, it was discovered that 114 fetal specimens remained at six places, with another one found later. These were all specimens of fetuses aborted in the sanatoria. It can be surmised that these fetal specimens were made from autopsies in order to prove placental infection.[6]

At Hansen's disease sanatoria, autopsy of aborted fetuses for placental infection study was carried out on a wide scale. At the 114th regular meeting of the Dermatology Society's Okayama region, Ōshima sanatorium director Kobayashi Wasaburō reported that "in cells from tissue samples of internal organs from the fetuses of leprosy patients, ranging from 3 months to 10 months, procured from recent induced miscarriages or still births," he had found leprosy bacilli, albeit only a few (Kobayashi 1929). Later in 1935 again at the Ōshima sanatorium, in 13 samples of placentas procured during the seven years from 1927, Inaba Toshio[7] examined them for leprosy bacillus (Inaba 1938). And in 1936 Muneuchi Toshio[8] searched to see whether or not there was leprosy bacillus in internal organs of 18 samples "procured from still born or artificially aborted fetuses of leprosy patients" (Muneuchi 1937).

---

1. 胎児標本　　2. 性感染症　　3. 野島泰治　　4.「生殖伝染」
5. 『ハンセン病問題に関する検証会議最終報告書別冊胎児標本調査報告書』　　6. 胎盤感染
7. 稲葉俊雄　　8. 宗内敏男

5. Eugenic Protection Law

As stated above, the eugenic idea of cutting off the descendants of the "inferior" clearly exists in the sterilization of Hansen's disease patients. Certainly it was an extermination policy[1] to cut off patients and their descendants.[*3] However, as long as it was denied to be a genetic disease, it could not be subject to the National Eugenics Law. The approval of the National Eugenics Law could mean that sterilization of leprosy patients would become illegal. On this issue, the Ministry of Health's Prevention Bureau Eugenics section director Tokonami Tokuji[2] said "concerning leprosy, a good reason can be permitted" (Tokonami 1941). His comment shows an attitude of acceptance of the continuation of sterilizing Hansen's disease patients outside the law (see Fujino 1993, 236-254).

The dissolution of these measures outside the law came in 1948. The National Eugenic Law was replaced by the Eugenic Protection Law[3] which specified the sterilization and abortion of Hansen's disease patients and their spouses. The members of the House of Councillors who were involved in creating the bill, Taniguchi Yasaburō[4] and Fukuda Masako,[5] gave the congenitally weak resistance to the disease as the reason for making Hansen's disease patients and their spouses subjects of the law (Taniguchi and Fukuda 1948). Again after the war, Mitsuda claimed that the sperm of male patients caused infection in the fetus and continued to cite this as the grounds for necessity of sterilization (Mitsuda 1952). Moreover, in a lecture given at a leprosy management workshop held at Nagashima Aisei-en on March 6, 1949, he emphasized the necessity of study of placental infection: there is

> the need to reverify the placenta from now on. I believe that the bacteria pass through the placenta. ... Because at the time when to speak of placental infection was mistakenly equated with heredity, we said it was postnatal infection without emphasizing placental infection. But today we should abandon such thoughts and research this problem more thoroughly. (Mitsuda 1950b)

Concerning this lecture, the director of Ōshima Seishō-en[6] (previously called Ōshima Sanatorium) Nojima Taiji, who advocated a genetic predisposition, reported that "in six out of fourteen cases of induced miscarriage, I have seen bacilli—in the ulnar nerve, lungs, liver, spleen, placenta, etc.—but it is unclear whether it is leprosy bacillus or not" (Mitsuda 1950b). It is clear that under the Eugenic Protection Law postwar autopsies of aborted fetuses were continued.

1. 絶滅策　　2. 床次徳二　　3. 優生保護法　　4. 谷口彌三郎　　5. 福田昌子
6. 大島青松園

Thus, under the Eugenic Protection Law after World War II for similar reasons as before the war, sterilizations and abortions were carried out on Hansen's disease patients (see Fujino 2006, 82-89). In 1951 Nagashima Aisei-en[1] conducted a nationwide survey of all of the National Leprosy Sanatoria (with the exception of those Okinawa and Amami) and the private sanatorium Minobu Shinkyō-en[2]. It was found that 1,397 couples had been sterilized; 561 couples had not been. The results show that 71.3% of the patient couples were sterilized ("Vasectomy in National Leprosarium" document at Nagashima Aisei-en). According to reports issued by the Labor Minister's Secretariat Statistical Information section "Yūsei hogo tōkei hōkoku" [Statistical report of eugenic protection] and "Botai hogo tōkei hōkoku" [Statistical report of maternal protection], the final sterilization commensurate with the provisions of the Eugenic Protection Law was conducted in 1992, and the last abortion in 1996. It is no exaggeration to say that the worst victims of eugenics policy in Japan were the Hansen's disease patients and their families.

Notes

*1 Formed in 1936, Unit 731 was formally called the Epidemic Prevention and Water Purification Department of the Kwantung Army. In the Harbin area they researched and produced chemical and biological weapons which were used in China. They also conducted experiments, including vivisections, on political prisoners and prisoners of war—many of whom died in those experiments.

*2 In a shocking article entitled "Kyū Kumamoto Ikadai Hansenbyō kokkaku hyōhon" [旧熊本医科大ハンセン病骨格標本 Former Kumamoto University Medical School Hansen's disease skeleton specimens] in the May 9, 2013 *Kumamoto Nichinichi Shinbun* [熊本日日新聞 Kumamoto Daily News], the morals of the doctors in the predecessor of the present Kumamoto University School Department of Medicine were brought into question.

*3 Concerning forced abortion and forced sterilization, Komatsu Hitoshi explains that the doctors who carried out the procedures gave as their reason "humanitarian action"—to prevent the patient's condition from worsening due to pregnancy. But he raises questions about whether that was medically valid and points out that the purpose was the "extinction of Hansen's disease patients" (see Komatsu 2007).

References

Fujino Yutaka [藤野豊]. 1993. *Nihon fashizumu to iryō—Hansenbyō wo meguru jisshōteki kenkyū* [日本ファシズムと医療—ハンセン病をめぐる実証的研究 Japanese fascism and medical care— demonstrative study about Hansen's disease]. Tokyo: Iwanami Shoten.

———. 2012. "Dai 15 kai Nihon raigaku sōkai ni okeru Ogasawara Noboru—Enshūji shozō

---

1. 長島愛正園　　2. 身延深敬園

'Ogasawara kankei monjo' no bunseki (1) ［第15回日本癩学総会における小笠原登―圓周寺所蔵「小笠原関係文書」の分析（1）Dr. Noboru Ogasawara in the 15th Japan leprology society general meeting—Analysis of "Dr. Noboru Ogasawara-related document" possessed in Enshuji temple (1)］in *Bulletin of Keiwa College* 21:2, 43-63.

―――. 2006. *Hansenbyō to sengo minshushugi—naze kakuri wa kyōsei sareta no ka* ［ハンセン病と戦後民主主義 Hansen's disease and postwar democracy—why was segregation forced?］. Tokyo: Iwanami Shoten.

―――. 2013."Kumamoto ni okeru 'Hansen byō kanja kokkaku hyōhon' mondai no kenshō"［熊本における『ハンセン病患者骨格標本』問題の検証 An examination of the 'skeletal specimens of Hansen's disease patients' issue in Kumamoto］in *Kikan sensō sekinin kenkyū* ［季刊戦争責任研究 Study of War Responsibility Quarterly］81 (Dec.), 62-65.

Hayashi Yoshinobu ［林芳信］. 1940. "Oyako oyobi dōho rai kanja no kansatsu"［親子及同胞癩患者の観察 Parent and child as well as fellow leprosy patients］Dai 13 kai Nihon Rai Gakkai gakujutsuenzetsu shōroku ［第一三回日本癩学会学術演説抄録 Excerpts of academic lectures at the 13th Japan Leprosy Society］in *Lepra* ［レプラ］11:1 (Jan.), 123-124.

Inaba Toshio ［稲葉俊雄］. 1938. "Raikanja taiban no byōri saikingakuteki kenkyū"［癩患者胎盤の病理細菌学的研究 A pathological bacteriological study of the placenta of lepers］in *Lepra* ［レプラ］9:5, 197-206.

Japan Law Foundation. 2005. "Verification Committee Concerning Hansen's Disease Problem Final Report (Summary Version)." 〈http://www.mhlw.go.jp/topics/bukyoku/kenkou/hansen/kanren/dl/4e.pdf〉

Kobayashi Wasaburō ［小林和三郎］. 1929. "Raikanja taiji no naizō zōkisoshiki nai ni okeru raikin"［癩患者胎児ノ内臓々器組織内ニ於ケル癩菌 Leprosy bacillus in the tissues of internal organs of the fetuses of leprosy patients］in *Hifuka oyobi hinyōkika zasshi* ［皮膚科及泌尿器科雑誌 Dermatology and Urology Journal］29:7 (July).

Komatsu Hiroshi ［小松裕］. 2007. "Hansenbyō kanja no sei to seishoku ni kansuru gensetsu no kenkyū"［ハンセン病患者の性と生殖に関する言説の研究 Study of statements about sexuality and reproduction of a Hansen's disease patient］in *Kumamoto journal of culture and humanities* ［熊本大学文学部論叢］93 (Mar.), 23-41.

Mitsuda Kensuke ［光田健輔］. 1906. "Raibyō kanja ni taisuru shochi ni tsuite"［癩病患者に対する処置に就て About the treatment of leprosy patients］in *Yōikuin geppō* ［養育院月報 Orphanage Monthly Bulletin］, 59. Mitsuda Kensuke to Nihon no Raiyobōjigyō ［光田健輔と日本の癩予防事業 Mitsuda Kensuke and prevention of Hansen's disease］, 29. Tokyo: Iwanami Shoten.

―――. 1930. "Sei no Dōtoku" ［性の道徳 The morals of sex］in *Yamazakura* ［山桜］12:6, 4-5.

―――. 1936. "'Wazekutomii' 20 shūnen" ［「ワゼクトミー」二十周年 20th anniversary of "vasectomy"］in *Aisei* ［愛生］6:4 (April), 48-54.

——— 1950a. *Kaishun Byōshitsu* [回春病室 Kaishun Hospital Room]. Tokyo: Asahi Shimbunsha.

——— 1950b. "Raibyōri kōshūkai kōen" [癩病理講習会講演 Leprosy management workshop lecture] in *Rai ni kansuru ronbun* [癩に関する論文 Papers about Leprosy] 3, 106-107.

——— 1952. "Thirty-five years of vasectomy" in *Leprosy in India* 23:3 (July), 127.

Muneuchi Toshio [宗内敏男]. 1937. "Raikanja no taiji ni okeru raikin no kensaku" [癩患者の胎児に於ける癩菌の検索 Search for leprosy bacillus in the fetuses of leprosy patients] in *Lepra* [レプラ] 8:1.

Nakajō Suketoshi [中條資俊]. 1934. "Rai densen no keiro ni tsuite" [癩伝染の径路に就テ About the process of leprosy contagion] in *Kōshūeisei* [公衆衛生 Public health] 52:6 (June), 11-15.

Nojima Taiji. [野島泰治]. 1932. "Raikanja no sei seikatsu oyobi hinin mondai" [癩患者の性生活及び避妊問題 Sex life of leprosy patients or contraception issues] in *Yuseigaku* [優生学 Eugenics], 108.

Suzue Kitasu and Nagase Toshiyasu [鈴江懐・永瀬寿保]. 1931. "Rai no honshitsuteki kenkyū (Dai ikkai hōkoku) [癩の体質的研究（第一回報告）The Essential Study of Leprosy (First Report)] in *Nihon Byōri Gakkai Kaishi* [日本病理学会会誌 Japan Society of Pathology Journal] 21, 143-144, 147.

Suzue Kitasu and Miyazaki Matsuki [鈴江懐・宮崎松記]. 1943. "Rai shishinzō ni okeru roima kessetsu ni tsuite" [癩屍心臓に於けるロイマ結節に就テ About rheumatoid nodules found in the hearts of leper's cadavers] in *Nihon Byōri Gakkai Kaishi* [日本病理学会会誌 Japan Society of Pathology Journal] 33, 119.

Suzue Kitasu [鈴江懐]. 1941. "Rai to Taishitsu" [癩と体質 Leprosy and Physical Constitution] in *Taishitsugaku zasshi* [体質学雑誌 Physical constitution studies magazine] 9:3 (Feb.), 319.

——— 1951. "Batsu ni kaete—Rai kenkyū no omoide to kore kara no kōsō [跋にかえて―癩研究の思い出とこれからの構想―Postscript—Memories of Leprosy study and ideas therefrom] in *Rai no byōri chiken hoi, sono ta* [癩の病理知見補遺，その他 Supplementary notes on leprosy pathology, etc.], ed. Suzue Kitasu, 53-55. Hifuka Kiyō Henshūbu.

Takashima Shigetaka [高島重孝]. 1939. "Rai no soshitsu to kateinai densen ni tsuite" [癩ノ素質ト家庭内伝染ニ就テ About the diathesis of leprosy and contagion in the home] in *Keiō igaku* [慶應医学] 19:11 (Nov.), 80.

Taniguchi Yasaburō [谷口弥三郎] and Fukuda Masako [福田昌子]. 1948. *Yūseihogohō kaisetsu* [優生保護法解説 Explanation of the Eugenics Protection Law]. Osaka: Kenshinsha.

Tokonami Tokuji [床次徳二]. 1941. "Kokumin Yūseihō ni tsuite" [国民優生法に就いて About the National Eugenics Law] in *Minzoku eisei* [民族衛生 Race hygiene] 9:1 (May), 58-66.

Ueki Tetsuya [植木哲也]. 2008. *Gakumon no bōryoku: Ainu bochi wa naze abakare ta ka* [学問の暴力―アイヌ墓地はなぜあばかれたか Academic violence: why was the Ainu cemetery violated?]. Yokohama: Shumpusha.

Epilogue

Karen J. Schaffner

Japan embraced eugenics when emphasis was being placed on the nation taking its rightful place as a member of the "civilized nations" of the world. Included in the civilization process were rapid industrialization, capitalistic economy, colonial expansion, and urbanization. Eugenics was seen as offering a solution to many of the resulting social problems. Some eugenic policies were patterned after those of other "civilized nations." Others were adopted in order to deal with conditions that were considered to be a national embarrassment in the eyes of other "civilized nations." Still others were implemented to ensure that Japan would have the human resources necessary for colonization and mobilization for war. Importing Western ideas, Japan selected and fashioned those ideas to meet its needs and situation. While it can be said that there were some benefits from sanitation measures, medical advances, and contagious disease control, related policies also required that the good of the state come before individual freedoms and rights. As Daniel Wikler comments about eugenics, "those who actually bore the brunt of state coercion in the name of the eugenic common sense were usually the marginal,[1] the stigmatized,[2] and the vulnerable"[3] (Buchanan 2000, 35). As in other countries, that was also the case in Japan.

Like eugenics in other countries, eugenics in Japan was promoted primarily by people of middle and upper classes. Starting motivations and methods were often quite different, but, in the end, some people were victimized. Eugenics also had a racial emphasis, and was linked with nationalism[4]—"interpreting the degeneracy thesis in national terms, identifying nationality with "blood" and fearing that England (or Germany, or wherever) would lose in competition with nations that did a better job maintaining the quality of their germ plasm" (Buchanan 2000, 34). Identifying degenerative traits and preventing them from being passed on future generations was important for protecting the national gene pool. A perusal of articles in *Yūseigaku* [Eugenics] reveals the idea that, regarding the national welfare, people with "undesirable" traits,[5] defective genes,[6] inherited diseases,[7] or disabilities[8] were con-

1. 社会の隅に置き忘れられた者　2. 汚名を着せられた者　3. 弱い者　4. 国家主義
5. 有害な形質　6. 欠陥のある遺伝　7. 遺伝病　8. 障害

sidered a burden or even a threat. Legislation was passed and policies put into place to lessen the burden and counter the threat.

When Japan lost in the "competition" of the Pacific War and began rebuilding its war-torn economy and society under American occupation, eugenics was still a part of this process. As Matsubara Yōko[1] indicates, the postwar Eugenic Protection Law[2] of 1948 targeted a broader base than the 1940 National Eugenic Law,[3] including measures for compulsory sterilization[4] with simplified procedures and approval of birth control[5] and abortion[6] (Matsubara 1998).

Discussing eugenics in America, Donald Pickens has maintained that the growth of a "belief in economic and environmental determinism," Hitler's eugenic excesses, and advances in genetics overturned the basic tenets of eugenics and resulted in its decline and rejection in the 1930s (Pickens 1968). But more recent studies suggest that eugenics did not just disappear. Science historian Garland Allen queried whether there "Is a New Eugenics Afoot" (Allen 2001), and sociologist Troy Duster spoke of a "back door to eugenics"—prenatal genetic screening[7] being one of those back doors (Duster 1990).

In his presidential address to the American College of Medical Genetics in 2003, geneticist Charles Epstein asks the question "is prenatal diagnosis eugenics?" He answers in this way:

... by the strictest definition—"eugenic" being equated with "well-born"—prenatal diagnosis is eugenics. But, ... from my point of view, prenatal diagnosis is, at worst, eugenics in name only, BUT!!... But, I would hope that we all agree that there is still much for us to think about with regards to what we are now doing, and even more to think about with regard to what we might be doing in the future—about carrier screening[8] before marriage, presymptomatic genetic testing,[9] preimplantation diagnosis,[10] gene therapy,[11] and the search for genetic components of behavior and intelligence" (Epstein 2003, 474-475).

Epstein's conclusion about eugenics has been critiqued by the disability rights community. Biology and ethics professor and activist Adrienne Asch, who had firsthand experience with disability, argued: "As currently practiced and justified, prenatal testing and embryo selection cannot comfortably coexist with society's professed goals of promoting inclusion and equality for people with disabilities" (Asch 2003, 315). The critique is based on three main points: prenatal diagnosis supports the idea that disability itself is not the problem, but society's discrimination against people with disability; it assumes that parents are unwilling to accept a child with disability; and it is based on

1. 松原洋子　2. 優生保護法　3. 国民優生法　4. 強制断種　5. 産児制限
6. 妊娠中絶　7. 出生前遺伝学的スクリーニング　8. 保因者スクリーニング
9. 発症前遺伝学的診断　10. 着床前診断　11. 遺伝子治療

misinformation about whether a child with disability can meet parental expectations. Questions also exist about whether genetic counseling[1] is truly non-directive and non-coercive and about whether the counselor contributes to societal discrimination that says not to have a capacity is grounds for terminating pregnancy. Asch says "having a capacity can be good, but the absence of capacity is simply an absence, it need not be seen as negative or 'dis-valuable'" (Asch 2003, 326).

An article in *The Japan News* (*Yomiuri Shimbun*) had as its headline—"98% opted for abortions after positive prenatal test" (Nov. 23, 2013, 2). Out of 3,514 Japanese women who took the test between April and December, sixty-seven tested positively for Down syndrome,[2] Trisomy[3] 13, or Trisomy 18. For six of these, further tests showed no abnormalities, though one gave birth to a child later diagnosed with Trisomy 18. Two had miscarriages before further tests could be done, and fifty-six chose to terminate their pregnancy, some citing not being confident they would be able to raise the child as the reason for their choice. Three chose not to undergo further tests.

Allen noted that "we seem to be increasingly unwilling to accept what we view as imperfection in ourselves and others" (Allen 2001, 61). There exists today, as there did in prewar eugenics, the tendency to measure the worth of a person's life on a cost-benefit basis:[4] how much of an economic and emotional burden will the person place on society and on the family, how much can the person contribute to society. As genetic research gives us more options for diagnosis, cures, and, perhaps someday, enhancement,[5] we have lessons to learn from the history of eugenics. We need to rethink what it means to live a meaningful life and how to make a better life for future generations.

Arai Eiko[6] considered these questions, drawing on her friendship with Hansen's disease patients and her own fight with cancer. Her reflections provide us with food for thought:

> When people make strength or size the basis of their bonds [with other people], right away efficiency is preferred, and the logic of exclusion is brandished. But when weakness is the basis for bonds, you notice that weakness has a mysterious power. It does not exclude anyone. It makes the most of each other's gifts…. And in a relationship where everyone is in the same position and doing the same things for each other, people forgive each other and offset each other's weakness, creating peace of mind and trust (Arai 2011, 48).

References

Allen, Garland E. 2001. "Is a New Eugenics Afoot?" in *Science* 294 (Oct. 5), 59, 61.

1. 遺伝カウンセリング　2. ダウン症候群　3. トリソミ　4. 費用対効果の観点
5. ［遺伝子による］能力増強　6. 荒井英子

Arai Eiko [荒井英子]. 2011. *Yowasa wo kizuna ni—Hansenbyō ni manabi, gan wo ikite* [弱さを絆に―ハンセン病に学び，がんを生きて― (Making) Weakness a bond: learning from Hansen's disease and living with cancer]. Tokyo: Kyobunkan.

Asch, Adrienne. 2003. "Disability Equality and Prenatal Testing: Contradictory or Compatible?" in *Florida State University Law Review* 30:2, 315-342.

Buchanan, Allen, et al. 2000. *From Chance to Choice: Genetics and Justice.* Cambridge: Cambridge University Press.

Duster, Troy. 1990. *Backdoor to Eugenics.* New York: Routledge.

Epstein, Charles J. 2003. "Is modern genetics the new eugenics?" in *Genetics IN Medicine* 5:6 (Nov.-Dec.), 469-476.

Matsubara Yōko. 1998. "The Enactment of Japan's Sterilization Laws in the 1940s: A Prelude to Postwar Eugenic Policy" in *Historia Scientiarum, The History of Science Society of Japan*, 8:2 (Dec.), 187-201.

Pickens, Donald K. 1968. *Eugenics and the Progressives.* Nashville, TN: Vanderbilt University Press.

Chronology of Eugenics in Japan

M: Meiji T: Taishō S: Shōwa H: Heisei

1868 M:1	• Meiji Restoration
1873 M:6	• 1. 1 Home Ministry (*Naimushō*) established • Japan participated in Austrian International Exposition in Vienna (5. 1-11. 1) • Franz M. Hilgendorf introduced evolutionary theory in his lecture at Tokyo Medical School
1874 M:7	• Aoigawa Nobuchika addressed evolutionary theory in *Kitagō dan* [Story of Northern Country]
1875 M:8	• 4. 19 Fukuzawa Yukichi's *An Outline of a Theory of Civilization* • 7. 25 Kyoto Insane Asylum established; first public mental hospital (abolished 1882)
1876 M:9	• 6. Erwin von Bälz arrived from Germany to teach at the Medical Academy of Tokyo
1877 M:10	• 4. 12 Tokyo University established • 10. 6 E. S. Morse lectured on evolution at Tokyo University for the public • Cholera epidemic; more than 100,000 victims
1878 M:11	• 10. 20 Formation of Biological Society of Tokyo University by Morse and Yatabe Ryōkichi
1879 M:12	• 4. 30 Matsubara Shin'nosuke wrote about Hilgendorf's evolution lecture in *Seibutsu shinron* [New Theory of Life] • 7. 25 Tokyo Insane Asylum established • Central hygiene committee created as a consultative body for mental hygiene (with Mori Arinori as president) and local commission set up in each prefecture
1881 M:14	• 7. Partial translation of C. Darwin's *Descent of Man and Selection in Relation to Sex* as *Jinsoron* [Ancestors of Man] by music educator Kōzu Senzaburō

	• 9. Fukuzawa Yukichi introduced F. Galton's *Hereditary Genius* in *Jijishōgen* [Commentary on current problems]
1882 M:15	• 2. 25 Botanical Society of Tokyo founded
1884 M:17	• Takahashi Yoshio proposed intermarriage of Westerners and Asians as strategy for race improvement in *Nippon Jinshu Kairyōron* [A Treatise on the betterment of the Japanese race] • Nagayo Sensai asserted marriage not only determines fate of individual but also that of future generations in *Kon'in heigairon* [Discussion of Marriage Abuse]
1885 M:18	• Zoological Society of Tokyo founded • Fukuzawa Yukichi's "Datsu a ron" [On departure from Asia]
1886 M:19	• 12. 6 Tokyo Woman's Christian Temperance Union (WCTU *Tokyo Kirisutokyō fujin kyōfū kai*) organized • Katō Hiroyuki criticized Takahashi's proposal in "Nippon jinshu kairyō no ben" [Discussion of the betterment of the Japanese race] • Fukuzawa Yukichi emphasized the importance of improving parents and the environment • Bälz' lecture on improvement of Japanese race, siding with Katō
1889 M:22	• 2. 11 Promulgation of the Greater Japan Imperial constitution • 9. Gotō Shinpei sets forth Darwin's theory of evolution as the principle for national hygiene in *Kokka eisei genri* [Principles of National Hygiene] • 10. 25 Izawa Shūji's complete translation of Thomas H. Huxley's *Origin of species: Or the Causes of the Phenomena of Organic Nature* as *Shinka genron* [The Principle of Evolution] • Japan exhibition at Paris Exposition
1893 M:26	• 4. 3 *Nihon Kirisutokyō fujin kyōfū kai* [Japan woman's Christian Temperance Union] organized
1894 M:27	• 4. 22-26 "Hygiene Specimen Exhibition" • 4. 12th Annual Meeting of Greater Japan Private Hygiene Association in Kyoto • 8. 1 First Sino-Japanese War (until 1895)

1896 M:29	• 3. 22 Tachibana Senzaburō's translation of Darwin's *The Origin of Species* as *Seibutsushigen ichimei genron* [The Origin of Living Things]
1900 M:33	• 3. 10 Mental Patients' Custody Act [*Seishinbyōsha kangohō*] • 3. Public Order and Police Law [*Chian keisatsu-hō*] prohibited women's participation in politics (abolished 1945. 11.) • 4. 1 *Miseinensha kitsuen kinshi-hō* [Law prohibiting the smoking of tobacco by minors] put into effect • 10. 2 Regulation for the Control of Prostitutes [*Shōgi torishimari kisoku*]
1901 M:34	• 5. 19 First socialist party organized—Social Democratic Party (prohibited on day after founding) • Kure Shūzō appointed chief of Sugamo Hospital of Tokyo prefecture
1903 M:36	• Kuwano Hisataka introduced Mendel's laws of heredity in *The Zoological Magazine* in a translation of A.D. Darbishire's article • Bulletin of Charity Association for the Help of Mental Patients', *Shinshitsusha no kyūgo* [Help for mental patients] published • "Anthropology Pavilion" at 5th Domestic Industrial Exhibition in Osaka
1904 M:37	• 2. 8 Russo-Japanese War (until 1905)
1905 M:38	• 4. 10 Fujikawa Yu began *Jinsei* [Life] magazine (continued until 1918. 12. 1)
1906 M.39	• 10. Abe Isoo's *Risō no hito* [Ideal person] • Toyama Kametarō demonstrated that heredity silkworms followed Mendel's law • Shimoda Utako *Joshi no eisei* [Female hygiene]
1907 M·40	• 3. 19 *Raiyobō ni kansuru ken* [Act on Leprosy Prevention] (enforced from 1909. 4. 1) • Penal code promulgated, human trafficking not specified as a crime • Ogata Masakiyo in *Fujin no katei eisei* [Women's home hygiene] summarized marriage hygiene
1908 M:41	• Greater Japan Civilization Society established to introduce Western learning

1909 M:42	• 12. 24 Kagawa Toyohiko began work in Kobe's Shinkawa slums • National sanatoria for segregation of Hansen's disease patients established in Osaka, Kagawa, Kumamoto, Tokyo, and Aomori
1910 M:43	• 4. Brothel licenses for Sonezaki pleasure district in Osaka terminated • 6. 20 Abe Isoo's *Fujin no risō* [Ideals of women] published • 8. 29 Annexation of Korea • Unno Yukinori published *Nihon jinshu kaizōron* [On remodeling the Japanese race]
1911 M:44	• 5. Oka Asajirō's *"Minshu kaizengaku no jissai kachi"* [The real value of ethnic betterment study] • Unsuccessful attempt to move Yoshiwara pleasure district in Tokyo from city center after fire (4. 9); *Kakuseikai* (Purity Society) organized to fight prostitution (7. 8) • Unno's *Kōkokusaku to shite no jinshu kaizō* [Race remodeling as a national policy]
1912 M:45 T:1	• 7. 15 Abe Isoo referred to "eugenics" in article "Nora and Magda"
1913 T:2	• 4. Tanaka Yoshimaro began first series of genetics lectures at Tohoku Imperial University • 11. Nagai Hisomu's lecture "Discussion of the Necessity for the Study of Racial Betterment—Eugenics"
1914 T:3	• 1. 3 Translation of C. Davenport's *Heredity in Relation to Eugenics*[*Jinshu kairyōgaku*]published by Greater Japan Civilization Society
1915 T:4	• 2. 12 Abe Ayao founded Japanese Society of Breeding • 11. 8 Kagawa's *Hinmin shinri no kenkyū* [The study of the psychology of the poor] • Mitsuda Kensuke began sterilization surgery on Hansen's disease patients at Zensei Hospital
1916 T:5	• 2. Galton's *Hereditary Genius* translated as *Tensai to iden* [Genius and Heredity] by psychologist Haraguchi Tsuruko • 7. Nagai Hisomu introduced sterilization in his book *Jinseiron* [Treatise on life]

| | • Research Committee for Health established
• Nationwide investigation of Hansen's disease in *burakumin* areas under Mitsuda Kensuke |
|---|---|
| 1917 T:6 | • 2. 16 Greater Japan Eugenics Society founded by Abe Ayao and Yamanouchi Shigeo |
| 1918 T:7 | • 4. Fujii Kenjirō taught first course of genetics at Tokyo Imperial University's Department of botany, endowed by Nomura Tokushichi and brothers
• Kure Shūzō and Kashida Gorō wrote report *Seishinbyōsha shitakukanchi no jikkyō* [Description and Statistical observation of the mentally ill under home custody] based on field study carried out 1910-1916 |
| 1919 T:8 | • 10. Matsuzawa Hospital established (originally Tokyo Insane Asylum)
• 12. Hiratsuka Raichō and members of the *Shin fujin kyōkai* (New Woman Association) prepared petition requiring men to be undergo premarital testing for venereal disease
• *Seishin byōin hō* [Mental Hospital Act] |
| 1920 T:9 | • 6. Japanese Society of Breeding reorganized as Genetics Society of Japan
• 12. Matsuzawa Hospital officially admitted under Mental Hospital Act
• Marriage Restriction against Men with Venereal Disease petition presented to Diet; unsuccessful but attracted attention in media |
| 1921 T:10 | • 5. Martin Barr lectured on "prevention of the feebleminded" at Psychiatry Conference in Tokyo, considering the legislation of sterilization
• Revised petition for premarital disease testing presented to Diet; also unsuccessful |
| 1922 T:11 | • 3. 10 Margaret Sanger visited Japan, increasing awareness of birth control; Yamamoto Senji issued translation of "Family Limitation" pamphlet
• 3. 30 *Miseinensha inshu kinshihō* [Juvenile Alcohol Prohibition Act] established
• 7. Baron and Baroness Ishimoto started Japan Birth Control Study Society
• 3. 25 Abe Isoo's *Sanji seigen ron* [Theory of Birth Restriction]
• Translation of P. Popenoe's and R. Johnson's *Applied Eugenics* [*Ōyō yūseigaku*] published by Greater Japan Civilization Society |

1923 T:12	• Yamamoto Senji started Birth Control Study group in Kansai; published *Birth Control Monthly* with Majima Yutaka
1924 T:13	• 1. 20 Gotō Ryūkichi founded *Nihon Yūseigakkai* [Japan Eugenics Society] • Charity Association for the Help of Mental Patients set up help station for earthquake victims • Kiyono Kenji's study of 52 skeletons excavated from Ainu tombs in Sakhalin • Tanaka Yoshimaro published *Ningen taishitsu no kaizen ga kyūmu* [The betterment of human physical qualities is urgent]
1925 T:14	• 2. 15 Yamamoto Senji started publication of *Sanji chōsetsu hyōron* [Birth control review]; title changed to *Sei to shakai* [Sex and Society] in October (continued until 1926 5. 25) • 3. Gotō Ryūkichi established monthly magazine of Japan Eugenics Society, *Yūzenikkusu* [Eugenics]; name changed to *Yūseigaku* in 1925 (continued until 1943. 3) • 4. 22 Promulgation of *Chian iji hō* [Peace Preservation Law] (enforced 5. 12, abolished 1945. 10) • 6. 1 Tanaka Yoshimaro published *Yūseigaku kara mita hainichimondai* [Anti-Japanese problem as seen from Eugenics]
1926 T:15 S:1	• 4. 15 Nakanomiya Hospital of Osaka Prefecture established under Mental Hospital Act • 10. *Sankōkan* [Archive] established on grounds of Japan Red Cross Headquarters in Tokyo's Shibadaimon • 11. 1 First issue of Ikeda's *Yūsei undō* [Eugenic Exercise/ Movement] magazine (continued until 1930. 1) • 11 Eugenic Exercise/Movement Association founded by Ikeda Shigenori
1927 S:2	• Charity Association for the Help of Mental Patients renamed *Kyūchi-kai* [Help Association] • 4. 5 Venereal Disease Prevention Law promulgated • 7. 7 Formation of Population Food Problem Investigation Committee
1928 S:3	• 5. 1-23 Ethnic Hygiene Exhibition held at Red Cross Museum • 12. Miyake Kōichi's "The characteristics of evil men observed from the psychiatric viewpoint" in *Yūseigaku*

	• Japanese Medical Association presented "Report to Home Minister about Race Hygiene"
1929 S:4	• 3. 5 Yamamoto Senji assasinated • 10. 31 Abe Isoo visited E. S. Gosney and P. Popenoe of Human Betterment Foundation in California • Kobayashi Wasaburō reported finding leprosy bacilli in autopsies of aborted and miscarried fetuses of patients • P. Popenoe's and R. Johnson's *Applied Eugenics* [*Oyō yūseigaku*] translated by Hara Sumitsugu
1930 S:5	• 11. 30 *Nippon Minzoku Eisei Gakkai* [Japan Society of Race Hygiene] founded by Nagai Hisomu • Abe Isoo translated E. Gosney's and P. Popenoe's *Sterilization for Human Betterment* as *Funin kekkon to ningen kaizō*
1931 S:6	• 1. 17 Birth Control League of Japan founded • 3. At 4th General Meeting of the Japan Leprosy Society discussion of inherited Hansen's disease criticized • 4. 2. Revised Act on Leprosy Prevention (Leprosy Prevention Law) • 4. Suzue Kitasu asserted predisposition to Hansen's disease based on study of patients' skulls • 6. Japan Association of Mental Hygiene established • 8. Lecture tour by R. Johnson sponsored by American Eugenics Society • 9. 18 Outbreak of "Manchurian Incident" • 12. 5 Abe Isoo's *Seikatsu mondai kara mita sanji chōsetsu* [Birth control seen from lifestyle problems] introduced sterilization as method of birth control • 12. Chikushi Sanitarium of Fukuoka Prefecture under Mental Hospital Act • Sanitarium of Kagoshima Prefecture (first built as a psychiatric ward of the Kagoshima Public Hospital in 1924) recognized as an independent institution
1932 S:7	• 7. 24 Formation of Social Mass Party • Japan Association of Mental Hospitals conducted census of Ainu in Hokkaido • Summer. Japan Society of Race Hygiene began investigation of the Ainu • Nojima Taiji insisted that abortion law or a contraception law was necessary for prevention of "reproductive contagion" of Hansen's disease

	• Red Cross Archive became Red Cross Museum (until 1963)
1933 S:8	• 6. 20 Eugenics marriage consultation center opened in Tokyo's Shiraki-ya Department Store by Japan Society of Race Hygiene • 11. 14−12. 17 Red Cross' *Kekkon eisei tenrankai* [Marriage Hygiene Exhibition] held jointly with the Japan Society of Race Hygiene • Eugenic marriage rules [*Yūsei Kon'in kun*]
1934 S:9	• 3. Ishimoto Shidzue opened Birth Control Consultation Center in Tokyo • 5. Japan Society of Race Hygiene excavated 131 complete skeletons from Ainu cemetery in Yakumo City Yūrabbu Beach • 6. E. Gosney and sterilization introduced in *Minzoku Eisei*; attempts begin to pass sterilization law • 7. Japan Society of Race Hygiene survey begun in Hokkaido village of Hiratori • 8. 5 Komai Taku *Nihonjin no iden* [Heredity of Japanese]
1935 S:10	• 2. Sterilization law draft *Nippon Minzoku Yūsei Hogohō* [Japanese Race Eugenic Protection Act] submitted to Diet; tabled • 11. 11 *Yūsei Kekkon Fukyūkai* [Eugenics Marriage Popularization Society] created by Japan Society of Race Hygiene • Japan Society of Race Hygiene attains foundation status and changes name to *Nihon minzoku eisei kyōkai* [Japan Association of Race Hygiene] (present name *Nihon minzoku eisei gakkai* [Japanese Society of Health and Human Ecology])
1936 S:11	• 5. Abe Isoo's "*Kokumin seikatsu to jinkō mondai*" [National life and the population problem] published • Mitsuda Kensuke purported theory that Hansen's disease is sexually transmitted
1937 S:12	• 7. 7 Second Sino-Japanese War (until 1945) • 12. 15 Ishimoto Shidzue arrested and interrogated about birth control activity and support of labor activist Katō Kanjū • 12 Kōfū-ryō of Hyōgo Prefecture established under Mental Hospital Act • Tuberculosis Prevention Ordinance
1938 S:13	• 1. Ishimoto ordered to close clinic and to cease all birth control activities • 1. Ministry of Health and Welfare established • 4. 22 First Racial Hygiene Conference; preparations made for passing

| | sterilization law
• 12. Kaneko Junji of Japan Society of Psychiatry and Neurology opposes Nagai's sterilization law
• Japan Society of Psychiatry and Neurology established an "Investigation Committee for Heredity" for psychosis cases |
|------|---|
| 1939 S:14 | • 9. Ministry of Health and Welfare's "The Ten Commandments of Marriage"
• 12. Oguma Mamoru promoted advancement of scholarship in *Kokuritsu idenkenkyūsho setsuritsu no kyūmu* [The urgent task of establishing a national genetics research institute],
• 12. 17 Abe Isoo spoke at meeting of Race Hygiene Group in Eugenic Division of Disease Prevention Department of Ministry of Health and Welfare, supporting sterilization
• *Nihon minzoku yūsei tenrankai* [Japan National Eugenics Exhibit] |
| 1940 S:15 | • 5. 1 National Eugenic Law enacted |
| 1941 S:16 | • 2. 22 Ogasawara Noboru's theory questioning the incurability and contagion of leprosy reported in *Chūgai Nippō*
• 7. 1 National Eugenic Law put into effect
• 11. 15-16 Ogasawara's comments suppressed and called mistaken
• 11. 17 "Joint Research of Leprosy" committee meeting affirmed Ogasawara's theory and need for discretion in reporting theory
• 12. 9 Outbreak of Pacific War following attack on Peal Harbor (12. 7) |
| 1943 S:18 | • 3. Help Association incorporated with Japan Association of Mental Hospitals and the Japan Association of Mental Hygiene to become *Seishin Kōseikai* [Association of Mental Welfare]
• Suzue reported on "leprosy allergy" based on autopsies of patients |
| 1944 S:19 | • Komai Taku criticized eugenics in *Idengaku sōwa* [Collection of genetics anecdotes]
• 5. Abe Isoo's *Kokumin no kakugo* [The preparedness of citizens] |
| 1945 S:20 | • 8. 15 End of Pacific War; U.S. occupation of Japan
• 11. Japan Socialist Party formed
• Mental Hospital of Kyoto Prefecture established under Mental Hospital Act |

1947 S:22	• 5. Institute of Genetics Foundation set up in Tokyo
1948 S:23	• 7. 13 Eugenic Protection Law [*Yūsei hogō hō*] (in force until 1996) • Since 1941, 538 persons sterilized under National Eugenic Law
1949 S:24	• 5. Kagawa Toyohiko's "Sanji chōsetsu ron" [On Birth Control] • 6. 1 National Institute of Genetics established • 8. 10 Oguma Mamoru became first director of National Institute of Genetics • 9. Clarence Gamble began financial contributions to Katō Shidzue for birth control activities and Koya Yoshio's "Three Village" birth control research projects
1950 S:25	• 5. 1 *Seishin eiseihō* [Mental Hygiene Act]
1951 S:26	• 9. 8 San Francisco Peace Treaty (U.S. occupation ends 1952) • Nagashima Aisei-en conducted a nationwide survey of National Leprosy Sanatoria
1952 S:27	• Koya Yoshio became head of Institute of Public Health • Mitsuda claimed sperm of males with Hansen's disease caused infection in fetus • 10. Margaret Sanger visited Japan, speaking against abortion and for population control
1953 S:28	• 3. Gamble met with leaders of various birth control groups, urging them to join forces, and join the International Planned Parenthood Federation • 8. 15 New Leprosy Prevention Law enacted • 9. Planned Parenthood Federation of Japan formed by merger of several groups
1954 S:29	• 4. 15 Margaret Sanger addressed Japanese Diet on population problems and family planning
1955 S:30	• 10. 24-25 Fifth International Congress of Planned Parenthood hosted in Tokyo by Planned Parenthood Federation of Japan
1961 S:36	• Yoshimasu Shūfu published *Yūseigaku* [Eugenics], insisting on heredity of mental illness and need for eugenics

1964 S:39	• 3. 24 U. S. Ambassador Edwin O. Reischauer stabbed in assassination attempt by released mental patient, resulting in call for revision of Mental Hygiene Act
1965 S:40	• 6. Mental Hygiene Act revised, abolishing "protective custody" and enforcing involuntary confinement
1972 S:49	• 5. 23 Revised Eugenic Protection Law proposed; *Aoi Shiba no Kai* began movement opposing amendment; bill was tabled and finally rejected
1984 S:59	• 3. Incident at Utsunomiya Hospital reported; death of mental patients brought international criticism of treatment
1987 S:62	• 9. 26 Mental Hygiene Act renamed Mental Health Act
1996 H:8	• 4. 1 New Leprosy Prevention Law abolished • 6. 18 Maternal Protection Law [*Botai hogohō*] replaced Eugenic Protection Law under which since 1948 some 16,500 persons had been compulsorily sterilized
2001 H:13	• 5. 11 Kumamoto court ruled policies for Hansen's disease patients unconstitutional • 6. State apology made to Hansen's disease patients • 6. 15 Law of Compensation for Hansen's disease patients

Index

Biographical Index

A

Abe Ayao（Fumio）［阿部文夫］（?-1945） 21, 29n, 72, 79n

Abe Isoo［安部磯雄］（1865-1949） 44-55, 76, 77

Agassiz, Louis［アガシー，ルイ］（?-1873） 16

Aoigawa Nobuchika［葵川信近］（?-?） 29n

B

Bälz, Erwin von［ベルツ，エルヴィン・フォン］（1849-1913） 7, 10

Bellamy, Edward［ベラミー，エドワード］（1850-1898） 46

Binding, Karl［ビンディング，カール］（1841-1920） 84

Boeters, Gustav［ベータース，グスタフ］（1869-1942） 84

C

Coleman, Elizabeth（Mrs. Horace E.）［コールマン，エリザベス］（18??-1932） 50

Coulter, John［コールター，ジョン］（1851-1928） 20

D

Darré, Richard-Walther［ダレ，リヒァルト＝ヴァルター］（1895-1953） 86

Darwin, Charles［ダーウィン，チャールズ］（1809-1882） 1, 15-17, 18, 83

Davenport, Charles Benedict［ダヴェンポート，チャールズ・ベネディクト］（1866-1944） 20, 71-73, 105, 112

de Vries, Hugo［ド・フリース，ユーゴ］（1848-1935） 17

F

Fujii Kenjirō 藤井健次郎（1866-1952） 17, 21

Fujikawa Yū［富士川游］（1865-1940） 37, 114

Fujimoto Sunao［藤本直］（?-?） 87

Fukuda Masako［福田昌子］（1912-1975） 137

Fukuzawa Yukichi［福澤諭吉］（1835-1901） 8-11, 17

G

Galton, Francis［ゴルトン，フランシス］（1822-1911） 1, 2, 6, 11, 15, 17, 18, 83, 105, 108

Gamble Clarence［ギャンブル，クラレンス］（1894-1966） 18, 79

Gosney, Ezra Seymour［ガスニー，エズラ・シーモア］（1855-1942） 50, 52, 74, 75, 77, 79, 112, 114

Gotō Ryūkichi［後藤龍吉］（1887-19??） 72, 73, 79, 107

Gotō Shinpei［後藤新平］（1857-1929） 98

Günther, Hans F. K.［ギュンター，ハンス

160 *Index*

F. K.］（1891-1968）　86

H

Haruguchi Tsuruko［原口鶴子］（1886-1915）　17

Hatoyama Ichirō［鳩山一郎］（1883-1959）　108

Hilgendorf, Franz Martin［ヒルゲンドルフ，フランツ・マルチン］（1839-1904）　16

Himmler, Heinrich［ヒムラー，ハインリッヒ］（1900-1945）　86

Hiratsuka Raichō［平塚らいてう］（1886-1971）　64, 66, 127, 128

Hitler, Adolf［ヒトラー，アドルフ］（1889-1945）　2, 50, 51, 86, 144

Hoche, Alfred［ホーヘ，アルフレート］（1865-1943）　84

Hoffmann, Géza von［ホフマン，ゲーツァ・フォン］（1885-1921）　84

Huxley, Thomas H.［ハックスリー，トマス・H.］（1825-1895）　16, 17

I

Ichikawa Fusae［市川房枝］（1893-1981）　127, 128

Ichikawa Genzō［市川源三］（1874-1940）　102

Ikeda Shigenori［池田林儀］（1882-1966）　17, 107

Ikeno Sei'ichirō［池野成一郎］（1966-1943）　18

Inaba Toshio［稲葉俊雄］（1908-1990）　136

Ishii Shirō［石井四郎］（1892-1959）　133

Ishikawa Chiyomatsu［石川千代松］（1860-1935）　16, 18, 19, 28n, 72

Ishikawa Tomoyoshi［石川知福］（1891-1950）　115

Ishimoto Shidzue［石本静枝］（1897-2001）（See Katō Shidzue）　77, 78

Izawa Jūji［伊澤修二］（1851-1917）　16

J

Johnson, Roswell Hill［ジョンソン，ロズウェル・ヒル］（1877-1967）　73-75, 79, 105

Juliusburger, Otto［ユリウスブルガー，オットー］（1867-1952）　84

K

Kagawa Toyohiko［賀川豊彦］（1888-1960）　45, 52, 123, 128

Kaneko Junji［金子準二］（1890-1979）　36, 40, 113

Kaneko Kentarō［金子堅太郎］（1853-1942）　10

Kaneko Tadakazu［金子直一］（?-1944）　73

Katayama Tetsu［片山哲］（1887-1978）　45

Katō Hiroyuki［加藤弘之］（1836-1916）　8, 9, 17, 112

Katō Kanjū［加藤勘十］（1892-1978）　77, 78

Katō Shidzue［加藤シヅエ］（1897-2001）　78

Kawamura Tamiji［川村多実二］（1883-1964）　22

Kikuchi Jin'ichi［菊池甚一］（?-1951）　38, 40, 113

Kimura Motoo［木村資生］（1924-1994）　27, 28

Kirihara Yasumi［桐原葆見］（1892-1968）　115

Kiyono Kenji［清野謙次］（1885～1955）　132, 133

Kodama Sakuzaemon［児玉作左衛門］（1895-1970）　125, 126, 132

Kobashi Ichita［小橋一太］（1870-1939）

100
Kobayashi Wasaburō［小林和三郎］（1881-1933）　134, 136
Komai Taku［駒井卓］（1866-1972）　23-26, 27, 72
Kōtoku Shūsui［幸徳秋水］（1871-1911）　45
Koya Yoshio［古屋芳雄］（1890-1974）　78, 79n, 80n
Kōzu Senzaburō［神津専三郎］（1852-1897）　16
Kure Shūzō［呉秀三］（1865-1932）　36, 39, 42

L
Laughlin, Harry Hamilton［ロフリン，ハリー・ハミルトン］（1880-1943）　71, 73, 79
Lenz, Fritz［レンツ，フリッツ］（1887-1976）　86

M
Majima Yutaka (Kan)［馬島佩］（1893-1969）　77, 78
Marui Kiyoyasu［丸井清泰］（1886-1953）　38
Matsubara Shin'nosuke［松原新之助］（1853-1916）　16
Matsumura Shōnen［松村松年］（1872-1960）　22
Mendel, Gregor［メンデル，グレゴル］（1822-1884）　8, 24, 27, 102
Mitsuda Kensuke［光田健輔］（1876-1964）　52, 54, 124, 125, 131, 132, 135, 137
Miyake Kiichi［三宅驥一］（1876-1964）　17
Miyake Kōichi［三宅鑛一］（1876-1954）　36, 37, 39, 41, 42
Miyazaki Matsuki［宮﨑松記］（1900-1972）　133

Morgan, Thomas Hunt［モーガン，トマス・ハント］（1866-1945）　23, 27, 105
Morse, Edward S.［モース，エドワード S.］（1838-1925）　7, 16, 18
Muneuchi Toshio［宗内敏男］（?-?）　136
Murata Masataka［村田正太］（1884-1974）　134, 135

N
Nakajō Suketoshi［中條資俊］（1872-1947）　134
Näcke, Paul［ネッケ，パウル］（1851-1913）　84
Nagai Hisomu［永井潜］（1876-1957）　21, 37, 39, 41, 64, 76, 108, 109, 112-115, 124
Nagayo Sensai［長興専齋］（1838-1902）　104
Naruse Jinzō［成瀬仁蔵］（1858-1919）　23
Nemoto Shō［根本止］（1851-1933）　62, 64
Niijima (Neesima) Jō［新島襄］（1843-1890）　44, 46
Nohara Moroku［野原茂六］（?-?）　21
Nojima Taiji［野島泰治］（1896-1970）　136, 137
Nitobe Inazō［新渡戸稲造］（1862-1933）　112

O
Ogasawara Noboru［小笠原登］（1888-1970）　135
Ogata Masakiyo［緒方正清］（1864-1919）　104
Oguma Mamoru［小熊捍］（1885-1972）　22-25
Oka Asajirō［丘浅次郎］（1868-1944）　19, 20, 106
Osawa Kenji［大澤謙二］（1852-1927）

114
Ōshima Hiroshi［大島広］(1885-1971)
  22

P

Pearl Raymond［パール，レーモンド］
  (1879-1940)　19, 29n
Popenoe, Paul Bowman［ポペノー，ポール・ボーマン］(1888-1979)　50, 52, 73, 75
Ploetz, Alfred［プレッツ，アルフレート］
  (1860-1940)　84, 86, 108

R

Rüdin, Ernst［リューディン，エルンスト］
  (1874-1952)　84, 86, 86

S

Sanger, Margaret Higgins［サンガー，マーガレット・ヒギンズ］(1879-1966)
  77-79
Shibata Keita［柴田桂太］(1877-1944)
  18
Shimoda Mitsurō［下田光造］(1885-1978)
  36, 38
Spencer, Herbert［スペンサー，ハーバート］(1820-1903)　1, 10, 15, 17
Suzue Kitasu［鈴江懐］(1900-1988)
  132, 133
Suzuki Zenji［鈴木善次］(1933-)　3, 9

T

Tachibana Senzaburō［立花銑三郎］(1867-1901)　17
Takahashi Yoshio［高橋義雄］(1863-1937)
  8-11
Takano Iwasaburō［高野岩三郎］(1871-1949)　37, 45
Takano Rokurō［高野六郎］(1884-1960)
  109
Takashima Shigetaka［高島重孝］(1907-1985)　134

Tanaka Yoshimaro［田中義麿］(1884-1972)　21, 22, 24-27, 106
Teruoka Gitō［暉峻義等］(1889-1966)
  114, 115
Taniguchi Yasaburō［谷口弥三郎］(1883-1963)　137
Thyssen, Fritz［ティッセン，フリッツ］
  (1873-1951)　86
Tokonami Tokuji［床次徳二］(1904-1980)
  137
Toyama Kametarō［外山亀太郎］(1867-1918)　18, 20-22

U

Uchida Kakichi［内田嘉吉］(1866-1933)
  108
Uematsu Shichikurō［植松七九郎］(1888-1968)　38, 40
Ujihara Sukezō［氏原佐蔵］(1884-1931)
  124
Unno Yukinori［海野幸徳］(1879-1954)
  106, 124

W

Wada Toyotane［和田豊種］(1880-1967)
  38
Wagner, Gerhard［ヴァーグナー，ゲルハート］(1888-1939)　86
Weismann, August［ヴァイスマン，アウグスト］(1834-1914)　18, 28n

Y

Yagi Takatsugu［八木高次］(1892-1944)
  115
Yakabe Ryōkichi［矢田部良吉］(1851-1899)　16
Yamakawa Kikue［山川菊枝］(1890-1980)
  77
Yamamoto Senji［山本宣治］(1889-1929)
  77, 78, 107
Yamanouchi Shigeo［山内繁雄］(1876-

1973） 20, 21
Yasuda Tokutarō［安田徳太郎］（1898-1983） 106
Yoshida Shigeru［吉田茂］（1885-1954） 23, 88, 108
Yoshimasu Shūfu［吉益脩夫］（1899-1974） 39, 41, 42

Topical Index

A

abortion［妊娠中絶 *ninshin chūzetsu*］ 27, 77, 78, 89-91, 116, 117, 136, 137, 138, 144

Act on Leprosy Prevention［癩予防ニ関スル件 *Raiyobō ni kansuru ken*］（1907） 131

adverse selection［逆淘汰 *gyaku tōta*］ 27, 28

Ainu［アイヌ］ 7, 99, 125, 133

alcohol［酒 *sake*, アルコール］ 61, 62, 66, 102/ alcoholics［アルコール依存症患者 *arukōru izonshō kanja*］ 48, 50, 52, 76, 84, 85, 89, 123, 124/ alcoholism［アルコール中毒, *arukōru chūdoku*］ 51, 87, 101

America（United States of） 1, 3, 6, 10, 16, 25, 39, 44, 46, 48, 50, 53, 61, 62, 71, 76, 78, 79, 84, 98, 105, 112, 122, 144

American Birth Control League［アメリカ産児制限同盟 *amerika sanji seigen dōmei*］ 71, 77

American Eugenics Society［アメリカ優生協会 *amerika yūsei kyōkai*］ 1, 71, 73

Aoi Shiba no Kai［青い芝の会］ 116, 117

Article 769 of the Civil Code［民法第769条］ 105

B

"Be fruitful and multiply"［産めよ殖やせよ Umeyo Fuyaseyo］（sometimes translated "Bear more, produce more" or "Propagate and multiply" 52, 53, 77, 89

bioethics［生命倫理 *seimei rinri*］ 3, 103, 118

birth control, birth restriction［産児調節 *sanji chōsetsu*, 産児制限 *sanji seigen*］ 47, 48, 50, 53, 55, 74, 77-79, 107, 108, 111, 117, 144

Botanical Magazine［植物学雑誌 *Shokubutsu-gaku zasshi*］ 16

Buraku Liberation Movement［部落解放運動 *Buraku kaihō undō*］ 123

burakumin［部落民］ 123, 125, 128n

C

California［カリフォルニア州 *kaliforunia shū*］ 75, 76, 112

capitalism［資本主義 *shihonshugi*］ 44, 46, 54

Caritas［カリタス karitasu］ 83, 85

Cold Spring Harbor Experimental Station［コールドスプリングハーバー実験所 *kōrudo supuringu hābā jikkensho*］ 29n, 71, 72

criminal［犯罪者 *hanzaisha*, 犯罪の］ 26, 40, 48, 50, 52, 76, 84, 90, 113, 123

E

epilepsy/ epileptic［てんかん *tenkan*］ 48, 72, 76, 85, 87, 90, 109

Eugenic Protection Law［優生保護法 *Yūsei hogōhō*］1948-1996 26, 40, 54, 90, 97, 117, 122, 137, 138, 144

Eugenics Record Office［優生記録局 *Yūsei kiroku kyoku*］ 10, 71-73, 118, 128

Eugenics Marriage Popularization Society［優生結婚普及会 *Yūsei kekkon fukyūkai*］ 65

Euthanasia Action［安楽死作戦 *Anrakushi sakusen*］（1939-1945） 84, 87

evolution/evolutional theory［進化論 *shin-*

karon] 6, 16, 18, 19, 39, 98

F

feebleminded [精神薄弱 seishinhakujaku] 39-41, 72-77, 85, 87, 89, 90, 101, 111

fukoku kyōhei [富国強兵 wealthy nation, strong army] 7, 15, 98

G

Genetics Society of Japan [日本遺伝学会 Nihon idengakukai] 18, 20-22, 24, 25, 27, 106

Germany [ドイツ doitsu] 3, 7, 36, 37, 39, 44, 46, 50, 51, 83, 87, 88, 90, 105, 108 112

"good wives, wise mothers" [良妻賢母 ryōsai kenbo] 61, 69

Greater Japan Private Hygiene Association [大日本私立衛生会 Dainippon shiritsueiseikai] 100, 101

H

Hansen's disease [ハンセン病 Hansen byō] 52, 77, 90, 102, 122-125, 131-133-138, 145

hereditary disease [遺伝病 iden byō] 41, 48, 49, 51, 55, 109

Home Ministry/Office [内務省 Naimushō] 35, 37, 38, 100, 112, 115, 118

Home Ministry Department of Public Health [内務省衛生局 Naimushō eisei kyoku] 38, 74, 124

Human Betterment Foundation [人間改良財団 Ningen kairyō zaidan] (1926-1944) 74-76, 79

human genome [ヒトゲノム hitogenomu] 28, 97

Hungtinton's Chorea [ハンチントン舞踏病 Hanchinton butōbyō] 51, 87

Hygiene exhibit [衛生展覧会 Eiseitenrankai] 100, 101

Hygiene Specimen Exhibition [衛生参考品展覧会 Eisei sankōhin tenrankai] 101

I

Indiana [インディアナ州 indiana shū] 75, 84

Inner Mission [内国伝道 Naikoku dendō] 83, 85

International Exposition [万国博覧会 Bankoku Hakurankai] 99

J

Japan Association of Mental Hygiene [日本精神衛生協会 Nihon seishin eisei kyōkai] 38

Japan Birth Control League [日本産児調節連盟 Nihon sanjichōsetsu renmei] 50

Japan Birth Control Study Society [日本産児調節研究会 Nihon Sanjichōsetsu Kenkyūkai] 77

Japan Eugenic Exercise/Movement Association [日本優生運動協会 Nihon yūsei undō kyōkai] 20, 22, 107

Japan Medical Association [日本医師会 Nihon ishi kai] 49

Japan National Eugenics Exhibit [日本民族優生展覧会 Nihon minzoku yūsei tenrankai] (1939) 103

Japan Socialist Party [日本社会党 Nihon shakai tō] 45, 128

Japan Society of Breeding [日本育種学会 Nihon ikushugakkai] 21

Japan Society of Psychiatry and Neurology [日本精神神経学会 Nihon seishin shinkei gakkai] 113

Japan Society of Race Hygiene [日本民族衛生学会 Nihon Minzoku Eisei Gakkai] 19, 20, 39, 65, 76, 102, 108, 112, 125

Japonism [ジャポニズム japonizumu] 99

K

kōhaku zakkon [黄白雑婚 *yellow-white mixed marriage*] 8
Kikuchikeifū-en [菊池恵楓園] 133
Kuryū-rakusen-en [栗生楽泉園] 134

L

Labor-Farmer Party [労働農民党 *Rodō nōmin tō*] 45
Law for the Prevention of Hereditarily Diseased Offspring (See Nazi Sterilization Law) [遺伝病子孫予防法 *Idenbyō shison yobōhō*] (1933-1945) 39, 50, 86, 87
leprosy [癩, らい *rai*] (see Hansen's disease) 37, 49, 66, 107, 104, 122, 124, 134, 135
Leprosy Prevention Law [らい予防法 *Rai yobōhō*] 90, 98, 131

M

Manchuria [満州 *Manshū*] 45
Marriage Hygiene Exhibition [結婚衛生展覧会 *Kekkon eisei tenrankai*] (1933) 102
Maternal Protection Law [母体保護法 *Botai hogohō*] (1996-) 90, 91, 117
Matsuzawa Hospital [松沢病院 *Matsuzawa Byōin*] 35-37
Mendel's law of heredity [メンデル遺伝法則 *Menderu iden hōsoku*] 8, 17-19, 34
Mental Hospital Act [精神病院法 *seishin byōinhō*] (1919) 35, 37-40
Mental Patients' Custody Act [精神病者監護法 *Seishinbyōsha kangohō*] (1900) 34, 35, 38, 39, 98
Mental Hospital Law [精神病院法 *Seishin byōinhō*] 35, 36
Mental Hygiene Act [精神衛生法 *Seishin eiseihō*] (1950) 35, 38
military comfort women [従軍慰安婦 *jyūgun ianfu*] 127, 128
Ministry of Education [文部省 *Monbushō*] 16, 17, 21, 25, 100, 135
Ministry of Health and Welfare [厚生省 *Kōseishō*] 35, 51, 39, 77, 89, 90, 102, 103, 108, 109, 113

N

National Genetics Research Institute [国立遺伝研究所 *Kokuritsu iden kenkyūjo*] 23, 25, 27
National Eugenic Law [国民優生法 *Kokumin yūseihō*] (1940-1948) 23, 24, 39, 52, 54, 77, 88, 89, 97, 109-111, 113, 118, 131, 144
National Sanatorium Nagashima Aisei-en [国立らい療養所；国立療養所長島愛生園 *Nagashima Aisei-en*] 52, 74, 138
Nazi Sterilization Law [ナチス断種法 *nachisu danshuhō*] (1933-1945) 39, 50-52, 86, 87, 90, 91
New Woman Association [新婦人協会 *Shin-fujin kyōkai*] 64, 127

O

Ōhara Social Problems Institute [大原社会問題研究所 *Ōhara shakai mondai kenkyūjo*] 114
Ōshima Seishō-en [大島青松園] 64, 137

P

Pacific War [太平洋戦争 *Taiheiyo sensō*] (see World War II) 36, 38, 45, 89, 144
population problem [人口問題 *jinkō mondai*] 41, 47, 48
Population Problems Research Institute [人口問題研究所 *jinkō mondai kenkyūsho*] 103
poverty/pauperism [貧困 *hinkon*] 44, 46, 47, 61, 77, 123, 124
prenatal diagnosis [出生前診断 *shusseizen shindan*] 128, 144, 145

Index

prostitution ［売春 baishun］ 61-64, 66, 83, 123, 126, 127

Purity Society ［廓清会 Kakuseikai］ 63, 127

Prussian Sterilization Bill ［プロイセン断種法案 Puroisen danshu hōan］ 85

R

race betterment/ improvement ［人種改良 jinshu kairyō］ 6, 8-11, 48, 51, 106, 112, 123, 124

racial poisons ［人種の毒 jinshu no doku］ 61, 64-66, 103

Red Cross Archive ［赤十字参考館 Sekijūji sankōkan］ 61, 66, 103

Red Cross Museum ［赤十字博物館 Sekijūji hakubutsukan］ 100

Regulation for the Control of Prostitutes ［娼妓取締規則 Shōgi torishimari kisoku］（1900）98, 126

Russo-Japanese War ［日露戦争 Nichirō sensō］（1904-1905） 7, 22, 45, 72, 106

S

schizophrenia ［早発性痴呆 sōhatsu seichihō, 精神分裂病 seishin bunretsubyō, 統合失調症 tōgō shicchoshō］ 51, 87, 109

segregation ［隔離 kakuri］ 48, 75, 79, 118, 124, 131, 134, 135

Sino-Japanese war（1894-1895, 1937-1945）［日清戦争, 日中戦争 nisshin/nicchū sensō］ 7, 22, 23, 45

Social Common People's Party ［社会平民党 Shakai heimin tō］ 45

social Darwinism ［社会ダーウィニズム shakai dāwinizumu］ 7, 8, 15-17, 20, 22, 83

Social Democratic Party ［社会民主党 Shakai minshu to］ 44

Social Mass Party ［社会大衆党 Shakai taishū tō］ 45

Social People's Party ［社会民衆党 Shakai minshū tō］ 45

social problem ［社会問題 shakai mondai］ 2, 46, 74, 83

socialism ［社会主義 shakaishugi］ 44, 46, 54

Sotojima Hoyo-in ［外島保養院］ 134

sterilization ［断種 danshu/ 不妊手術 funin shujutsu/ 優生手術 yūseishujutsu］ 2, 26, 39-42, 47-53, 55, 74-77, 79, 83-85, 89-91, 103, 108, 109, 112-115, 122-124, 131, 132, 135-138, 144

T

Ten Commandments for Strengthening the Nation ［民族強化十訓 Minzoku kyōka jūsoku］（1939） 103

Ten Commandments of Marriage ［結婚十訓 Kekkon jūkkun］（1939） 102

tobacco ［タバコ tabako/ 喫煙 kitsuen］ 61, 62, 66

Tokyo Matsuzawa Hospital ［東京府立松沢病院］ 39

tuberculosis ［結核 kekkaku］ 37, 61, 66, 98, 101-103, 107, 114, 122

U

Unit 731 of the Japanese Imperial Army ［陸軍731部隊 Rikugun nana san ichi butai］ 133, 138n

V

vasectomy ［精系結紮 seikei kessatsu］ 49, 138

venereal disease ［性病 seibyō, 花柳病 karyūbyō］ 37, 64-66, 98, 101, 102, 111, 122, 126, 127

Venereal Disease Prevention Law ［花柳病予防法 Karyūbyō yobōhō］（1927） 127

Verification Committee Concerning Hansen's

Disease Problem Final Report［ハンセン病問題に関する検証会議最終報告書 *Hansenbyō mondai ni kansuru kenshōkaigi saishūhōkokusho*］　136

W・Y・Z

World War I［第一次世界大戦 *Dai ichiji sekai taisen*］　36, 77, 83, 84, 98, 123, 124

World War II［第二次世界大戦 *Dai niji sekai taisen*］　24, 90, 97, 118, 128, 138

Yamato race［大和民族 *yamato minzoku*］　7, 22, 107, 125

Zensei Hospital［全生病院 *Zensei byōin*］　124, 125, 131, 134

Eugenics in Japan（日本の優生学）

2014年6月30日 初版発行

編　者　カレン・J. シャフナー

発行者　五十川　直行

発行所　一般財団法人　九州大学出版会
〒812-0053 福岡市東区箱崎7-1-146
九州大学構内
電話　092-641-0515(直通)
URL　http://kup.or.jp/
印刷・製本／大同印刷㈱

Ⓒ Karen J. Schaffner 2014　　ISBN978-4-7985-0128-4

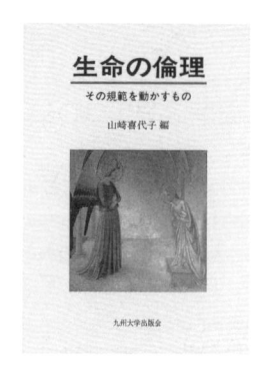

生命の倫理──その規範を動かすもの──

山崎喜代子 編　　A5 判・328 頁・2,800 円

ヒトゲノム解読計画が完了し，本格的なゲノム科学の時代を迎えている今日，これまでの生命倫理学規範である権利概念の限界を含めて，生命倫理学の構造的見直しを試みるとともに，時代の政治的経済的動機によって翻弄されてきた生命倫理規範の歴史を振り返る。

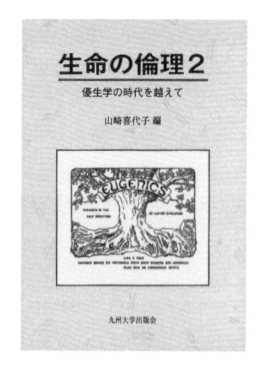

生命の倫理 2──優生学の時代を越えて──

山崎喜代子 編　　A5 判・352 頁・3,000 円

本書は，優生学とその政策を，諸科学・各国優生学・女性・衛生安全思想といった多様な切り口で分析する。さらに優生学時代を確実に乗り越えた，精神医学・胎児診断・臨床試験倫理など現代医療倫理の構築を試みるものである。

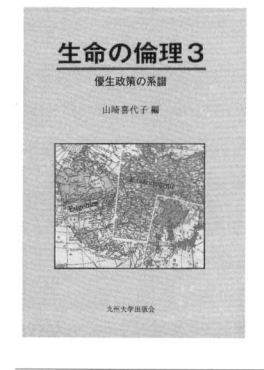

生命の倫理 3──優生政策の系譜──

山崎喜代子 編　　A5 判・450 頁・定価 3,200 円

優生学の政策化は 19 世紀の米国において開始され，戦前の日本においてもアジア進出に伴い政・軍・学を通して進められた。本書では欧米諸国の優生政策の成立と，戦前・戦中期の日本優生学の展開を解説する。19 世紀以降，今日までの優生学年表も収録。

(価格税抜)　　　　　　　　九州大学出版会